Palliative Care in Cardiac Intensive Care Units

Massimo Romanò

Editor

Palliative Care in Cardiac Intensive Care Units

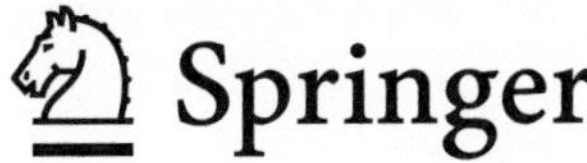

Editor
Massimo Romanò
Organizing Committee, Postgraduate
Master In Palliative Care
University of Milan
Milano
Italy

ISBN 978-3-030-80114-4   ISBN 978-3-030-80112-0   (eBook)
https://doi.org/10.1007/978-3-030-80112-0

This Springer imprint is published by the registered company Springer Nature Switzerland AG
The registered company address is: Gewerbestrasse 11, 6330 Cham, Switzerland

Foreword

Currently, Cardiac Intensive Care Units (CICU) provide care for people who are older, more frequently multimorbid and suffering from chronic, progressive diseases, both cardiac (chronic heart failure in particular) and non-cardiac, causing more complex health-related problems than in recent decades. The increasing accessibility of often invasive, advanced diagnostic procedures and treatment strategies implies challenging dilemmas with regard to the optimal allocation of resources and the selection of methods offering the prolongation of good quality life. The solution of such dilemmas requires care which addresses all components determining the quality of life (such as symptom management, including those caused by concomitant, non-cardiological diseases, support in the psychosocial and spiritual dimensions) as well as open and sensitive in-depth communication. This approach takes into account patients' personal goals and values, but also the risk of deterioration and death, being a prerequisite of shared decision-making. The inclusion of health care professionals with palliative care expertise in the multi-professional heart team can be supportive for patients and their relatives, but also for members of cardio teams.

As this book deals with palliative care for people admitted to the CICU, it focuses on the end stage of heart failure (i.e. stage D according to American College of Cardiology/American Heart Association) and people with a shortened life span/high risk of dying. It is important, however, to be aware that it is just a part of whole spectrum of palliative care that should be provided to all people living with a progressive disease (including heart failure) and who have health care needs that can be addressed by palliative care, irrespective of the stage of disease, predicted life span/risk of dying or planned treatment. With such a broad understanding of modern palliative care, limiting its provision only to those at risk of dying is inappropriate. The guidelines for the diagnosis and treatment of heart failure of European Society of Cardiology recommend the early introduction of palliative care, and its increase as the disease progresses. For the twenty-first century medicine, optimal disease-specific treatment and optimal symptomatic management should be mandatory at every stage of disease progression. The way to achieve this goal requires care for people living with heart disease provided in parallel by both disciplines—cardiology and palliative care. Depending on current needs, local traditions and the skill of health professionals, palliative care needs can be met using primary palliative care (i.e. the palliative care approach) or specialist palliative care.

The order of palliative care interventions presented in this book guides the reader from addressing the needs of *high urgency* (management of symptoms causing significant suffering if ineffectively treated, such as dyspnoea, pain or depression), through addressing more *chronic problems* (management of other symptoms, for example gastrointestinal) to more important ones as *psychosocial issues*, including decision-making. There are, however, dimensions that go beyond the classical medical service, sometimes mentioned as elements of palliative care, having the *highest meaning* for the individual person related to existential, transcendental and spiritual issues. Effectively addressing these needs, starting with those of greater urgency, opens up a space to realize and address those of greater significance.

Progress in cardiovascular medicine, especially in biotechnology, has improved the quality and/or length of life of many people with cardiovascular disease. However, devices (e.g. implantable cardioverter defibrillator, ICD, or mechanical circulatory support, MCS) not only influence the trajectory of life, but also of dying. If they remain fully active in the terminal phase of life, their continued functioning can be seen rather as preventing natural dying and prolonging life, after it has inevitably lost its quality and dignity, than as saving life. For this reason, after recognizing the approaching death, modification of their activity should be communicated (if this has not happened earlier, as recommended) and carried out. This decision is often challenging for patients, relatives and the care team. The primary objective underlying the rationale for treatment withdrawal must always be to respect the patient's right to live, or at least to die with dignity, by limiting any therapeutic action that increases the patient's level of stress, pain or anxiety. The discontinuation of futile therapies should be considered as a way to ensure the best quality of life and care, even during the final phase of life.

If the disease itself or the discontinuation of treatment causes suffering that persists despite optimal symptom management, palliative sedation should be considered and discussed with the patient. If it is approved, controlled administration of a drug causing limitation of consciousness and having a sedative activity (e.g. benzodiazepines, propofol or, less commonly in cardiological patients, dexmedetomidine) should be considered. To relieve other symptoms like pain or dyspnoea, parallel treatment with opioids may be necessary. Support for relatives beyond the dying phase and immediate interventions facilitating bereavement should be provided in these situations.

Providing the modern palliative care to people with heart failure who need it, together with optimal cardiological management, maximizes the possibility of allowing them as long a life as possible with the best possible quality.

Piotr Sobanski
Palliative Care Unit and Competence Centre, Spital Schwyz
Schwyz, Switzerland

EAPC Task Force on Palliative Care for People
with Heart Disease (2014–2021)
Vilvoorde, Belgium

Preface

I am a clinical cardiologist and for most of my professional life, now more or less 40 years, I have been taking care almost exclusively of patients with acute cardiovascular disease.

In the last ten years the world of cardiology units, including my own unit, has profoundly changed. These changes have mainly occurred in the clinical and epidemiological characteristics of patients admitted to cardiac intensive care units (CICUs): care has shifted from patients with acute coronary syndrome to elderly patients with a high prevalence of non-ischaemic cardiovascular diseases and non-cardiovascular comorbidities.

Both increase the susceptibility of patients to develop life-threatening critical conditions, which are associated with a significant burden of symptoms, length of stay and mortality rate. In this context, according to specific guidelines from scientific societies, palliative care programmes, including withholding/withdrawing life-sustaining treatments or deactivation of implanted cardiac devices, are often necessary.

However, discussing palliative care in the CICUs still appears to many cardiologists as an oxymoron, a contradiction in terms, because the training of physicians is aimed at always fighting death, even when this is no longer feasible.

Accordingly, all available technologies should therefore be used to achieve this goal, even though patients with a poor prognosis or deteriorating quality of life will receive little clinical benefit from intensive care, in the face of the high associated costs, both in terms of monetary expenditure and human suffering.

Consequently, the recommendations of scientific societies to implement the palliative care approach in clinical practice are still inconsistent. One of the main reasons for this gap is the cultural lag of cardiologists, who are not trained to deal with end-of-life care issues.

This book was born from these reflections, with the aim of spreading the culture of palliative care also in the world of acute cardiovascular care. The authors involved in it are among the most expert opinion leaders in their specific fields. All aspects of palliative care as applied to CICU are analysed, from epidemiological issues, to shared decision-making, to symptom control, all of which require formal education on end-of-life care.

Special attention is given to ethical issues, such as withholding/withdrawing life-sustaining treatments, deactivation of implanted cardiac devices, do not attempt resuscitation orders, and palliative sedation.

Finally, a special chapter highlights the relationship between ethics and technology in CICU, aware that the correct use of all advanced technologies should be used by applying the criteria of proportionality and appropriateness of treatments: this is the only way to implement the right tech/right touch philosophy.

I am confident that this book will help cardiologists, anaesthesiologists, palliative care specialists, nurses and all those involved in critical care to decide what is best for the patient and family in the advanced stages of cardiovascular disease.

Special thanks to Dr. Donatella Rizza, Executive Editor at Springer, with whom I have already shared successful publishing initiatives and who accepted this book proposal with her special usual enthusiasm, and to Aruna Sharma and Vignesh Manohar for their editorial assistance.

Milano, Italy   Massimo Romanò

Acknowledgements

The volume editor wishes to thank the Italian non-profit organization "Presenza Amica" for the financial contribution to the translation.

"Presenza Amica" is committed to protecting the dignity of patients in the advanced and evolving stages of illness, including chronic, oncological and non-oncological diseases with an unfavourable prognosis, and to supporting their families.

https://www.presenzamica.it/

Contents

About the Author

Massimo Romanò is a cardiologist, and he worked for 40 years in the Italian National Health System. From 1999 to 2003, he has been Head of Cardiac Electrophysiology in Garbagnate Milanese Hospital, Italy, and from 2003 to 2016 Head of Division of Cardiology in Vigevano Hospital (Pavia). This is a medical facility equipped with Cardiac Intensive Care Unit, Cath-Lab, EP-Lab and others. Since 2013, he is a member of the Organizing Committee of Postgraduate Master in Palliative Care, University of Milan. During the early 2000s he developed a particular interest in advanced heart failure and in end of life issues. He has been involved in the drafting of Italian position paper on shared care planning in end-stage chronic organ failures. He published many papers on palliative care issues in cardiac intensive care units and on the deactivation of implanted cardiac devices at the end of life. He has been the editor of the first Italian book dedicated to Palliative Care in Heart failure. He published two books on Clinical Electrocardiography edited by Springer.

Epidemiology and Patterns of Care in Modern Cardiac Intensive Care Units

1

Gianni Casella, Laura Sofia Cardelli, and Rodolfo Francesco Massafra

1.1 Introduction

Since the late 1960s, coronary care units (CCUs) have been developed to care for patients with acute myocardial infarction (AMI). Within these CCUs, well-trained and equipped staff offers accurate monitoring and prompt resuscitation in case of life-threatening arrhythmias [1, 2], and could prevent adverse events, including cardiac arrest. Furthermore, technological innovation promoted further conceptual shifts of CCU to the emerging field of critical care cardiology. The developments of reperfusion therapies (pharmacological or mechanical) in ST-segment elevation myocardial infarction (STEMI) and early revascularization for non-ST-segment elevation acute coronary syndromes (ACS) have contributed to a marked reduction in morbidity and mortality due to AMI. Later on, these benefits were further extended by the implementation of STEMI networks [3–5] where CCUs with interventional facilities are clearly the hub. Over the last decades, the traditional role of CCU has expanded to care for a broader spectrum of acute cardiovascular diseases (CVD), like acute heart failure (AHF), cardiogenic shock, unstable valvular heart disease, high-grade heart blocks, major ventricular arrhythmias, cardiac arrest, massive pulmonary embolism, cardiac tamponade, aortic dissection, devices infections, or complications of invasive procedures as well [6–12]. Moreover, as the population is aging and prevalence of noncardiac comorbidities increasing, CCUs often admit patients with cardiac complications of acute noncardiac diseases and the management of these

G. Casella (✉)
UOC di Cardiologia, Ospedale Maggiore, Azienda USL di Bologna, Bologna, Italy
e-mail: gianni.casella@ausl.bologna.it

L. S. Cardelli · R. F. Massafra
UOC di Cardiologia, Azienda Ospedaliera-Universitaria di Ferrara "Arcispedale Sant'Anna",
Cona (FE), Italy
e-mail: crdlsf@unife.it; mssrlf@unife.it

M. Romanò (ed.), *Palliative Care in Cardiac Intensive Care Units*,
https://doi.org/10.1007/978-3-030-80112-0_1

subjects could be challenging [13, 14]. Therefore, the definition of CCU has evolved to a more comprehensive "cardiac intensive care unit" (CICU) [6, 8, 15, 16]. Furthermore, development of advanced diagnostic or therapeutic technologies has claimed for an upgrade of the competence of cardiologists, with the rise of sub-specialized figures like electrophysiologists, interventional cardiologists, heart failure or imaging specialists, and intensive care cardiologists as well [7, 17–19]. All these changes have been clearly summarized within the Position Paper on the CICU organization and competencies issued by the Acute Cardiac Care Association (ACCA) in 2018 [20]. This paper addresses the different complexity of critical cardiac patients through a patient-oriented model. Thus, starting from clinical risk stratification of any individual acute cardiac patient, the correct level of care needed for a particular case is identified taking into account his/her clinical status, comorbidities, and available facilities [21]. The final result would triage individual patients to the correct level of care according to a three-level CICU's models, as described below. The functional role of each center within a hospital network is defined by its facilities and skillfulness in the treatment of specific critical conditions, allowing transfer of patients to higher or lower standards of care when their level of risk changes [22, 23], according to the principles of the "hub-and-spoke" model.

Therefore, along with ACCA indications the functional three-level system of care for CICU is defined as follows (Table 1.1):

1. Level I: CICUs are dedicated to the treatment of acute cardiovascular pathologies at risk of deterioration that need an intensity of care not available in a cardiology ward. These cases need continuous ECG and noninvasive hemodynamic monitoring, and may request noninvasive ventilation, intravenous inotropes and/or vasodilators, as well as immediate resuscitation of cardiovascular arrest. Level I CICUs mainly manage patients with medium- to low-risk non-ST-segment elevation ACS, congestive heart failure, and complex arrhythmias not at risk of deterioration. Within inter-hospital network for STEMI level I CICUs represent the peripheral "spoke" of this model of care where patients could be initially diagnosed or triaged to the hub, and referred back after reperfusion. In addition, if in close cooperation with a higher level CICU, level I CICUs can provide post-cardiovascular surgery monitoring, and they might act as step-down units of level II or III CICUs.

2. Level II CICUs are usually the hub of a STEMI network with immediate access to a 24 h/7 days coronary interventional catheter laboratory. Furthermore, they focus on severe AHF and patients with low cardiac output complicating other cardiac conditions. They must provide a more intensive level of monitoring, like central venous access, arterial line positioning, temporary transvenous pacing, percutaneous cardiac assist device (intra-aortic balloon pump or percutaneous axial pumps), and pericardiocentesis. They should be able to offer temporary invasive ventilation, with staff trained in its use.

3. Level III CICUs refer to complex acute cardiovascular conditions demanding a very critical care level of monitoring and intervention. These include extracorporeal circulatory support, invasive mechanical ventilation, renal replacement therapy (RRT), and emergent heart surgery. Level III CICUs constitute the top reference hospital for acute cardiovascular care in a particular

Table 1.1 Intensive cardiovascular care units' characteristics (modified from reference [20])

	Level I CICU	Level II CICU	Level III CICU
Population and disease	Non-ST-segment elevation ACS, hemodynamic stable congestive heart failure, complex arrhythmias not at high risk, monitoring of patients' post-structural and endovascular interventions	STEMI and high-risk ACS, severe or high-risk patients with congestive heart failure and/or low cardiac output complicating acute or chronic cardiac conditions	Mainly level III patients, some level II patients; acute cardiac conditions needing invasive mechanical ventilation, renal replacement therapy, ECLS, emergent heart surgery, or surgical cardiovascular assistance
Technology and therapy in CICU	• All noninvasive clinical parameters' monitoring • 24/7 Echocardiography and thoracic ultrasound; direct current cardioversion; noninvasive ventilation; transcutaneous temporary pacing	• All invasive and noninvasive cardiovascular monitoring • Idem level I CICU plus: Ultrasound-guided central venous line insertion; transvenous temporary pacing; transesophageal echocardiography; pulmonary artery catheter/right-heart catheterization; percutaneous circulatory support; X-ray system for fluoroscopy	• All advanced invasive and noninvasive cardiovascular monitoring • Idem level II CICU plus: Extracorporeal life support; mechanical circulatory support; renal replacement therapy; mechanical ventilation
Hospital	• Emergency department; CT scanner; transesophageal echo; X-ray system for fluoroscopy	• 24/7 Coronary interventional cath lab; hub center of a STEMI network • Idem for level I CICU plus pacing, cardiovascular resynchronization therapy; implantable cardioverter-defibrillator program; ablation therapy; renal support therapy; scanner and CMR	• Tertiary or university hospital • Idem for level II CICU plus percutaneous structural heart intervention; endomyocardial biopsy; donor organ and transplantation program; interventional vascular radiology; comprehensive cardiovascular surgery

(continued)

Table 1.1 (continued)

	Level I CICU	Level II CICU	Level III CICU
Level of competence	• Head: Cardiologist • Team: Cardiologists • On-site: Intensivist consultation 24/7	• Head: Cardiovascular intensivist • Team: Cardiovascular intensivists • On-site: Intensivist consultation 24/7	• Head: Cardiovascular intensivist or co-directorship with a general critical care specialist • Team: Cardiovascular intensivists with additional education in critical care; may include general intensivists with additional education in cardiology
Education programs	• Recommended: Written exam of the ESC-ACC certification for individuals; should master all the techniques required in level I CICU • Residents or fellow in cardiology	• Required: Specific national curriculum for acute cardiovascular care or ACCA curriculum for cardiovascular intensivist • Residents or fellow cardiovascular intensive care	• Idem level II CICU plus specific curriculum for general critical care training • Residents and fellow cardiovascular intensive care; critical care
On-duty physicians	• Cardiologists with level I CICU expertise; if approved by the unit's director, trained residents or other physicians provided availability of an on-call member of the CICU team	• Cardiovascular intensivists; trained cardiologists; physicians advanced in their cardiovascular intensivist training provided availability of a cardiovascular intensivist or an interventional cardiologist	• Should have all the requirements and expertise for working in a level III CICU
Nursing/ other personnel	• Nursing director (could be shared with regular ward) • Dedicated nurses—nurse-to-patient ratio 1:4	• Nursing director • Dedicated nurses—nurse-to-patient ratio 1:2 or 1:3	• Nursing director • Dedicated nurses—nurse-to-patient ratio 1:2 or 1:1
Research	• Encouraged to be part of outcome research	• Encouraged to conduct clinical research	• Strong commitment to perform clinical research

geographical area. They should be part of a university institution with resident or fellow training programs and should perform clinical and translational researches.

Notably, as complexity of CICU increases, the competence of cardiologists working within these units should evolve to a cardiovascular intensivist level with advanced training in critical care [24–26]. Furthermore, it is mandatory to develop close relationships with other subspecialties of cardiology and other medical specialties, like cardiovascular surgery and anesthesiology, nephrology, infectiology, clinical pharmacology, nutrition, and palliative care as well [27, 28]. To gather all these specialists, heart teams' organization models should be implemented to improve decision-making and routine discussion of complex cases [29].

Therefore, modern CICU should be considered a patient-oriented setting, where highly competent doctors and nurses master high-tech medicine with a strong attitude to networking and multidisciplinary care.

1.2 Is There a Background for the Evolution of CICU? From the Blitz-3 to Modern International CICU Registries

The demonstration of this perceived evolution from CCU to CICU had to wait long, until the publication in 2010 of the Italian Blitz-3 Registry [30]. This multicenter, prospective, observational study enrolled 6986 patients admitted to the 332 Italian CICUs during a 2-week time window in 2008. Patients observed were mainly elderly men (39% older than 75 years). Seventy percent had chronic comorbidities. ACS, mainly STEMI, accounted for 52% of all CICU admissions. Several other patients were admitted for non-ACS acute cardiac diseases. In particular, 14% of subjects were admitted for AHF, 7% for bradyarrhythmias, while pulmonary embolism, aortic dissection, and myocarditis were rather rare. Patients admitted to CICU were most often triaged from the emergency room (ER) and 18% of them had been brought to hospital through the emergency medical system (EMS). An echocardiogram was performed in 78% of cases. Interestingly, 4% of the patients needed temporary pacing and 3% electrical cardioversion, once the procedures that boosted the concept of intensive cardiac care units. Overall, ventilation, intra-aortic balloon pump, and ultrafiltration were rarely used. However, more than 90% of patients had at least a diagnostic or therapeutic procedure performed during their CICU stay. Almost 20% of the patients received insulin and 4% were transfused. The most common complications observed were new onset or worsening of heart failure and cardiogenic shock, but 11% of patients had a significant worsening of their renal function and 0.4% had a major bleeding as well. Median length of stay was 4 days (IQR 2–5) and the crude, in-CICU mortality of the overall population was 3.3%. Thus, the Blitz-3 Registry underlined a general change of epidemiology as compared to historically CCU, with a consistent aging, increases of non-ACS conditions cared, and complex interventions needed.

Patients admitted for STEMI (21% of the admissions) were younger and had a lower risk profile than the general population. Direct admission to CICU from EMS was observed in 61% of cases. Coronary angiography was performed in 65% of patients and 60% received reperfusion (15% fibrinolysis and 45% primary percutaneous coronary intervention). Counterpulsation was applied to 5% of patients and temporary pacing in 2%. The in-CICU, crude mortality of STEMI patients was 5.1%. Non-ST-segment elevation ACS was the most frequent cause of admission in CICU (31%): these patients were older and had a worse risk profile than the STEMI subjects. Only 35% of these cases were admitted to CICU through the ER. Coronary angiography was performed in 50% of cases and 32% were treated with percutaneous coronary intervention (PCI). Ventilation and counterpulsation were rarely used, but the most common complications observed were heart failure and angina or recurrent ischemia.

AHF accounted for 14% of the admissions. These patients were the oldest and had the worst risk profile. None of them was directly admitted to CICU through EMS; 79% underwent a transthoracic echocardiogram and 14% needed ventilation while in CICU. Only 10% of the patients underwent coronary angiography, and ultrafiltration, counterpulsation, electrical cardioversion, or temporary pacing was rarely necessary. The in-CICU, crude mortality of AHF was 5.4%.

Other acute non-ACS, non-AHF cardiac diseases accounted for 34% of the admissions. In this heterogeneous population, shock, heart failure, and arrhythmias were the most common complications, but length of stay was 1 day less and CICU crude mortality was lower (2.6%).

Interestingly, a secondary analysis of the registry assessed the distribution and level of appropriateness of hospital admissions according to the type of CICU. Hospital admissions for ST-segment elevation ACS occurred more frequently in type II or III CICUs ($p < 0.0001$), whereas type I facilities admitted more AHF subjects ($p < 0.0001$). Type I CICUs admit more patients not undergoing reperfusion ($p < 0.0001$) or treated with thrombolytic therapy ($p < 0.0001$), while primary PCI was performed more frequently in type II and III CICUs ($p < 0.0001$). Similarly, patients hospitalized for ACS underwent coronary angiography ($p < 0.0001$) and PCI more frequently in type II and III CICUs ($p < 0.0001$). Prevalence of low-risk rather than intermediate- or high-risk patients was higher in type I CICUs ($p < 0.05$). Thus, the Blitz-3 Registry demonstrated that resource availability preselects patients and could impact acute cardiac care if networking is not firmly pursued [31].

In summary, the Blitz-3 Registry confirmed that in 2008 ACS was still the main reason for admission, but numbers of AHF or acute non-ACS, non-AHF cardiac diseases, as well as comorbidities were substantial.

Few years later, Roubille et al. conducted a nationwide administrative analysis on 277,845 patients consecutively admitted to all the French CICUs [32]. Demographic characteristics of subjects enrolled were pretty similar to those of the previous Italian Registry [30] (median age: 71 years (IQR 59–81) in France vs. 72 years (IQR 61–80) in the Italian survey). Similarly, ACS cases were younger and male gender prevalence was higher as compared to AHF patients. Admission rates for ACS were comparable (49.0% vs. 52% in Italy), while primary admissions for

AHF were lower (10% vs. 14% in the Blitz-3). However, when AHF was accounted as primary or secondary diagnosis it was observed in 27.8% of cases. Global mortality rate was higher (4.5%) than that observed in the Blitz-3 Registry (3.3%). However, it must be noted that the Italian survey had a shorter follow-up, limited to the CICU stay, while Roubille et al. observed the entire hospital stay.

Importantly, the French Registry reported a substantial increase of direct admissions from the EMS to the catheterization laboratory bypassing the emergency room (47.5% in France vs. 4% in the Italian survey), reflecting the strong implementation of STEMI networking that occurred at the end of the first decade of 2000 in Europe.

In summary, the French Registry reports increasing numbers of AHF admissions and a further implementation of STEMI networking. Unluckily, due to the administrative nature of the study a detailed analysis of the population was not available and this limits the comparison of the French Registry with others.

Later on several other experiences, mainly from the other side of the ocean, were reported. Unluckily, these reports were mainly focused on AHA level I units comparable to level III ACCA CICU. Watson et al. analyzed 2193 consecutive patients admitted from January 1, 2015, to December 31, 2017, in AHA level I critical intensive care units (CICU) in the USA [33]. Patients admitted to level I CICU in the USA were in their sixties (median age: 67 years, 43% at least 70 years older). They had a high burden of comorbidities [diabetes (33%), chronic kidney disease (27%), chronic pulmonary disease (22%), and active malignancy (13%)] or chronic cardiac conditions [heart failure (46%), ischemic heart disease (41%), and atrial fibrillation (30%)]. Due to CICU complexity the main reasons for admission were shock/hypotension (26%), cardiopulmonary arrest (11%), and primary arrhythmia without arrest (9%). To note unlike European Registries, in this case ACS was the seventh most common reason for admission (7%). Several patients were managed with mechanical ventilation (36%) and 45% with pharmacological hemodynamic support. Acute renal replacement therapy was used in 7.6% of patients. A total of 12% of patients had pulmonary arterial catheters and 55% of patients had central venous and/or arterial lines. Of patients with cardiogenic shock, 28% received mechanical circulatory support (MCS). The median duration of stay was 2.9 days (IQR 1.4–5.7). In-hospital mortality was 17.6%, which reached 41.9% in cardiac arrest and 31.7% in shock. These data clearly underline the differences between the epidemiology of the highest level CICU and that observed in previous European studies where all the different CICU levels were considered together.

Soon later, other North American researches became available but all of them referred to the highest level CICUs. Bohula et al. [34] published data on 3049 consecutive patients admitted between September 2017 and September 2018 in a network of 16 US and Canadian AHA level I CICUs. Patients enrolled were younger than the European ones (median age: 65 years, 39% older than 70 years), with a significant burden of comorbidities [diabetes (34.8%), chronic kidney disease (24.1%), chronic pulmonary disease (14.2%), active malignancy (6.6%), ischemic heart disease (41.6%), and chronic heart failure (36.2%), as well]. Admission for ACS accounted for 31.8% (46.3% of which were STEMI), lower than that observed in the European registries but with large variability between centers (15–57%). Heart failure and/or cardiogenic shock accounted for 18.6% of admissions, but when heart failure was considered as secondary diagnosis its prevalence raised to 41.3%. In addition, AHF was associated with a higher burden of care than ACS (32.9% vs. 23.6% of the 13,923 CICU patient-days overall, longer hospitalizations, more procedures). Since the indications for admission in CICU were mainly respiratory failure (26.7%) and shock (21.1%, one-third being non-cardiogenic or mixed) this analysis underlined the need of broader knowledge and expertise on advanced ventilation or hemodynamic support when dealing with the highest level CICU. On the other side, even in this high-tech center, several patients were admitted only for observation and monitoring (36.2% overall, 13.6% of them for post-procedural observation). These findings are quite surprising since it is not worth to admit uncomplicated cases in very-high-tech environments. Finally, global in-CICU mortality rate was 8.3%, with wide inter-center variability (from 4.0% to 19.7%) and overall in-hospital mortality rate of 10.9%. However, the highest mortality rates were observed among patients admitted after cardiac arrest (45.3%), or neurologic emergencies (30.6%), but also patients with respiratory failure (24.1%) or cardiogenic shock (30.6%) and in need for continuous renal replacement therapy (CRRT) (34.5%) or for MCS (26.6%) had very high mortality rates.

Goldfarb et al. [35] published a retrospective study, analyzing patients admitted to a US academic center from January 2011 to December 2016. In this study, 6967 patients referred to the AHA level I CICU were compared with 10,892 patients admitted to the medical intensive care unit (MICU) of the same hospital. Patients admitted for postoperative care were excluded. CICU patients were older (70.5 vs. 66.2 years) and had more ischemic heart disease and hypertension and a lower burden of chronic comorbidities such as chronic renal insufficiency, chronic obstructive pulmonary disease, and diabetes. Although the proportion of admission for non-cardiovascular diagnosis was lower in CICU (21.4% vs. 89.2%), the prevalence of non-cardiovascular disease was substantial also in this setting. Moreover, intensity of critical care was higher in MICU, but still considerable in CICU. In fact, mechanical ventilation (12.7% CICU vs. 34.5% MICU), vasopressors or inotropes (24.5% CICU vs. 31.3% MICU), RRT (4.7% CICU vs. 10.2% MICU), and blood transfusion (15.5% CICU vs. 32.5% MICU) were needed less frequently in CICU than in MICU. However, the authors conclude that a high level of non-cardiovascular critical care competencies is needed also in CICU settings.

Finally, the study from Jentzer et al. [36] added further information because the authors analyzed 15,947 patients admitted between January 2007 and April 2018 to a single AHA level 1 CICU. Median age was 67.6 years, and it did not vary significantly over time. During the decade there was a global reduction in admission for ACS (from 44.1% in 2007–2009 to 40.3% in 2016–2018 overall, no change for STEMI, from 20% to 16.7% for non-ST-segment elevation ACS). There was a substantial increase of other cardiovascular diagnoses like AHF (from 30.8% to 61.2%), arrhythmias (ventricular arrhythmias increased from 14.2% to 31.9%, atrial fibrillation from 28.4% to 45.6%, complete heart block from 5.2% to 11.4%), or valvular heart disease (from 26.5% to 47%). Similarly, an increase was observed in shock diagnosis (from 7.4% to 23.8%), cardiac arrest (from 6.8% to 12.6%), respiratory failure (from 16% to 36.3%), and sepsis (from 5.3% to 15.1%) as well. Prevalence of organ dysfunction near-doubled (from 29.8% to 59.4%) and proportion of multiorgan failure was three times higher (from 12% to 34.6%). A growth was observed in the use of any invasive line (from 36.1% to 57%), vasopressors and inotropes (from 23.6% to 27.4%), mechanical ventilation (from 23.6% to 31.2%), and RRT (from 1.8% to 3.2%). By contrast, use of invasive coronary angiography and PCI declined (respectively from 59.4% to 52.4% and from 39.5% to 25.3%). In-hospital length of stay increased (from 7.4 to 8.3 days), but no change was observed for the one in-CICU. Overall hospital mortality did not change (unadjusted OR per year 1.01, 95% CI 0.99–1.03, $P > 0.1$), but after multivariable adjustment there was a decrease in mortality for those with any critical care diagnoses (adjusted OR per year 0.91, 95% CI 0.85–0.96, $P = 0.002$).

A comparison of the main features of the above studies is provided in Tables 1.2, 1.3, and 1.4.

In summary, these American data show that there is a strong overlap between the highest level CICU and a conventional intensive care unit since complex patients in critical conditions often share common features. In fact, also critical acute cardiac diseases have associated multiorgan failures that need ventilation, hemodynamic assistance, or aggressive multiorgan treatment.

Correct risk stratification becomes essential to improve CICU care. In fact, aging, increased comorbidity rates, and risk of futility urge proper triage and better allocation of resources in the contemporary CICU setting. Thus, it is not surprising why interest toward prognostic scores has increased substantially in recent years. Unluckily these risk scores are derived from the MICU experience, where they are already used successfully, and could not describe effectively CICU complexity.

A recent study by Bennett et al. [37] evaluated 10,004 patients admitted from 2007 to 2015 to an AHA level I CICU, comparing Acute Physiology and Chronic Health Evaluation (APACHE) IV score with APACHE III score and Oxford Acute Severity of Illness Score (OASIS), the only one validated in CICU to date [38]. APACHE IV score performed better than the others [predicted in-hospital mortality, with a receiver-operator characteristic (AUROC) curve of 0.82 as compared to APACHE III score (AUROC 0.81) and OASIS score (AUROC of 0.79)], although it had poorer calibration. Furthermore, APACHE IV reliably predicted use and length of noninvasive ventilation (respectively $P < 0.001$ and $P = 0.02$), as well as the burden of comorbidities (Charlson Comorbidity Index: $P < 0.001$).

Another study analyzed 9961 patients admitted to an AHA level I CICU from 2007 to 2015 and validated the prognostic accuracy of the simple Sequential Organ Failure Assessment (SOFA) score in contemporary CICU [39]. The score, which is easy to calculate, was assessed within 24 h from the admission and predicted in-hospital mortality with an AUROC of 0.83 (no significant difference compared to APACHE III and APACHE IV scores). In particular, a SOFA score lower than 2 predicted a low hospital and post-discharge mortality. In addition, the SOFA score demonstrated an incremental predictive power when obtained during hospitalization. However, in another study the performance of the SOFA score was suboptimal.

Table 1.2 Main causes of admission and outcomes in CICU

	BLITZ-3 Registry [30] ($N = 6986$)	Roubille et al. [32] ($N = 277,845$)	Watson et al. [33] ($N = 2193$)	Bohula et al. [34] ($N = 3049$)	Jentzer et al. [36] ($N = 12,418$)	Goldfarb et al. [35] ($N = 6967$)
Study year	2008	2014	2015–2017	2017–2018	2016–2018	2011–2018
Settings	332 Italian CICU (types I–III)	All French CICU (administrative data)	USA, type III CICU network	USA and Canada, type III CICU network	USA, type III CICU network	USA, type III CICU network
Population age, years [median (IQR)]	72 (61–80)	71 (59–81)	67 (55–77)	65 (55–75)	68	70
Age >75 years (%)	39	42	NA	NA	NA	NA
Male gender (%)	64	63	57	63	60	61
Acute coronary syndrome (%)	52	49	7	31.8	40.3	18.4
Heart failure (%)	14	10	8	18.6	61.2	8.4
Shock/hypotension (%)	6	NA	26	21.1	23.8	1.6
Cardiac arrest (%)	1	0.5	11	8.7	12.6	NA
Respiratory insufficiency (%)	NA	NA	17	26.7	36.3	3.7
PA (%)	9	NA	9	17	NA	12.6
NCD (%)	2	NA	17	22.7	NA	20.4
Length of stay in CICU, days [median (IQR)]	4 (2–5)	2 (1–4)	2.9 (1.4–5.7)	2.2 (1.1–4.5)	2.4[a]	1.8 (1–3.3)
Mortality (%)	3.3	4.5	17.6	8.3	6	4.8

CICU cardiac intensive care unit, *ACCA* Acute Cardiac Care Association, *IQR* interquartile range, *PPO* post-procedural observation, *PA* primary arrhythmias, *NCD* noncardiac disease, *NA* not available

[a]Mean value (SD ± 2.8)

Table 1.3 Main non-cardiovascular diseases in CICU

	BLITZ-3 Registry [30] ($N = 6986$)	Roubille et al. [32] ($N = 277,845$)	Watson et al. [33] ($N = 2193$)	Bohula et al. [34] ($N = 3049$)	Jentzer et al. [36] ($N = 12,418$)	Goldfarb et al. [35] ($N = 6967$)
Respiratory insufficiency (%)	14	NA	22	14.2	19.2	NA
Kidney disease (%)	8	NA	27.2	24.1	21.9	22
PVD (%)	14[a]	NA	13.5	9.4	5.4	NA
Infection/ sepsis (%)	1	0.2	NA	NA	15.1	2.2
Liver disease (%)	NA	NA	NA	3.2	2.7	4.5
Active cancer (%)	6	NA	12.9	6.6	20.1	1.6
Anemia (%)	7	NA	NA	NA	46.1	NA
Diabetes (%)	25	NA	32.5	34.8	29.2	11
CVD (%)	[a]	NA	8.3	9.8	10.5	3.8

CICU cardiac intensive care unit, *PVD* peripheral vascular disease, *CVD* cerebrovascular disease, *NA* not available

[a]In Blitz-3 Registry PVD and CVD are accounted together

Table 1.4 Main procedures used during hospitalization in CICU

	BLITZ-3 Registry [30] (N = 6986)	Roubille et al. [32] (N = 277,845)	Watson et al. [33] (N = 2193)	Bohula et al. [34] (N = 3049)	Jentzer et al. [36] (N = 12,418)	Goldfarb et al. [35] (N = 6967)
Coronary interventions	24	36	NA	NA	25.3	NA
Any mechanical ventilation (%)	4	0	36	21.4[a]	31.2	12.7
MCS (%)	1	NA	18.2	9.5	7.7	2.8
RRT (%)	1	NA	7.6	8	3.2	4.7
IVV/I/V (%)	8	NA	45	36.2	27.4	24.5
Invasive hemodynamics (%)	0.5	NA	12	11	19.7	NA

CICU cardiac intensive care unit, *MCS* mechanical circulatory support, *RRT* renal replacement therapy, *IVV/I/V* intravenous vasopressors/inotropes/vasodilators, *NA* not available

[a]Bohula series referred to invasive ventilation

Median mortality rate predicted by SOFA score was strikingly lower than the observed crude in-hospital mortality, showing poor calibration [34].

Jentzer et al. elaborated a novel prediction model for in-hospital mortality in the modern CICU environment: the Mayo CICU Admission Risk Score (M-CARS) [40]. The score was developed on patients admitted to an AHA level I CICU between 2007 and 2018, whose baseline characteristics, admission diagnosis, mortality, and complications rates are similar to those observed in current third-level CICU. M-CARS score ranges from 0 to 10 points, stratifying patients into a low risk (score <2; hospital mortality <1%), intermediate risk (score 2–4), and high risk (score >4; hospital mortality >50%). It is based on seven variables obtainable at the time of CICU admission (cardiac arrest, shock, respiratory failure, Braden skin score, blood urea nitrogen, anion gap, and red blood cell distribution width). The model, tested on a cohort of 10,004 patients and then validated on 2634 prospective patients, showed a good performance (AUROC of 0.86 for in-hospital mortality with a fine calibration) ($p = 0.21$).

In conclusion, prognostic scores could help stratification in CICU. APACHE III, APACHE IV, and SOFA scores have very good discrimination for overall hospital mortality. Discrimination was better for patients <70 years of age as compared to older ones ($p < 0.01$ by DeLong test) [41]. Although we should admit the limitations of current available scores, they could facilitate the identification of patients at their extreme or in conditions that could not benefit from aggressive treatments. In fact, futility and palliative care have both become important issues in CICU. Today, we should admit that intensive care improves survival, but does not always offer a better quality of life. Furthermore, sometimes CICU care could end up as futile, increasing physical, emotional, and economic burdens to patients and caregivers. In CICU, patients are often faced with difficult decisions and could experience high emotional burden. Thus, physicians should remember that the respect for patient's autonomy remains fundamental, as the right to decline treatment when perceived disproportionate to the benefits. Therefore, specific scores could add objective evidence to clinical judgment and help decision-making. These could be particularly useful when the issue is turning down aggressive therapies in favor of palliative care.

In the last decades, we have witnessed a large shift in CICU demographics. The increasing severity and changing nature of critical illness in CICU have blurred the lines that historically separated the CICU from other general or disease-specific intensive care units [4, 42]. Data derived from the level III CICUs are not immediately transferable to lower level units, but they mirror how cardiology for acute patients is evolving [43]. In the USA level III CICUs (level I AHA) are turning down ACS admission in favor of AHF or others, as opposed in Europe where ACS is still the main cause of hospitalization [30, 32]. This heterogeneity and the forthcoming epidemiological changes reinforce the importance of broader knowledge and skills in general cardiovascular medicine and critical care medicine for clinicians working in modern CICU [33–36]. This is particularly evident in level III CICUs where the main indications for hospitalization are respiratory and/or renal failure, systemic infections, and shock [34–36]. Thus, cardiac intensivists, i.e., physicians trained in both cardiology and critical care medicine, have emerged as a potential staffing solution to address the need for comprehensive critical care skills and expertise [25].

1.3 Aging, Comorbidity, and the Risk of Futility in CICU

In recent years the average age of patients receiving CICU care has increased, with rise in number of elderly patients through all the CICU settings [44]. Patients over 70 years of age have higher mortality, disease severity, and number of comorbidities as compared to the younger ones. Moreover, care of these elderly has to consider associated geriatric conditions (like multi-morbidity, polypharmacy, cognitive decline, delirium, and frailty) that could be exacerbated or destabilized by hospitalization in CICU. Therefore, assessment of frailty in the CICU although still not standardized could be very helpful. As already mentioned, several studies indicate that frailty assessment helps in shared decision-making, often leading to plans to minimize therapeutic risks, and to pursue targets on quality of life instead of survival goals [45, 46]. The intrinsic association of acute cardiovascular diseases with geriatric complexities implies a need for tailored approaches that interconnect these different domains [47]. Thus, CICU clinicians should individualize treatment plans by incorporating multidisciplinary assessment, management strategies, patients' wills, and awareness of multi-morbidity, polypharmacy, cognitive limitation, and frailty impact on care. All these caveats call for a strong mindset evolution of cardiac intensivists.

1.4 The COVID-19 Tsunami and Its Effect on CICU

The COVID-19 pandemic has presented a major, unheralded stress on the health systems because it has largely crushed workforce, organizational structure, systems of care, and critical resource supplies as well. During the first months of the COVID-19 pandemic to fight the growing number of cases and the need of more beds of intensive care units the hospital system has been reengineered. In fact, hospital structures and even hospital networks have been deeply reorganized to ensure provider safety, to maximize efficiency, and to optimize patient outcomes. CICU and critical care cardiologists have been particularly involved since they are uniquely positioned. In fact, these structures and physicians have large medical and intensive competencies that could be used to treat respiratory and cardiovascular complications of SARS-CoV-2 patients. Furthermore, they could support clinicians without critical care training who may be suddenly asked to care for these critically ill patients. Thus, in high-penetration areas like Northern Italy or elsewhere, cardiology departments have been deeply influenced. The number of beds of intensive care unit has been increased, and some hospitals have been totally dedicated to the care of COVID-19 patients. Elective procedures and interventions have been stopped, and several level I CICUs have been converted into COVID-19 intermediate care units. Regional AMI networks have been reengineered and treatment of STEMI patients has been centralized in level II CICU to guarantee primary PCI for most patients with STEMI and revascularization for moderate- to high-risk non-ST-segment elevation ACS patients. On the other hand, several level III CICUs turned down ACS cases to direct their high-tech skillfulness toward COVID-19 patients in need of mechanical ventilation or MCS support. Therefore, during the COVID-19 pandemic CICUs demonstrate very high flexibility due to their broad spectrum of competencies [48].

1.5 Conclusions

In conclusion, following the evolution of epidemiology and patterns of care of patients admitted modern CICU has moved away from the old CCU model. Today, CICUs have to face increasingly complex problems and need to virtuously allocate the great variety of resources and technologies available to the right patient. Furthermore, since the risk profile of the population is changing, with an increasing number of elderly with multiple noncardiac comorbidities, we should not be surprised if a strong overlap between the contemporary CICUs and traditional medical intensive care units arises. These changes call for an evolution of the clinical competencies of intensive care cardiologists as well. Furthermore, these competencies should take into account problems like acute and chronic pain, frailty, palliation, and end of life, once considered as nuances in the "old" CCUs.

References

1. Julian DG. Treatment of cardiac arrest in acute myocardial ischaemia and infarction. Lancet. 1961;2:840–4.
2. Lown B, Fakhro AM, Hood WB Jr, Thorn GW. The coronary care unit. New perspectives and directions. JAMA. 1967;199(3):188–98.
3. Fuster V. 50th anniversary historical article. Myocardial infarction and coronary care units. J Am Coll Cardiol. 1999;34:1851–3.
4. Van de Werf F, Bax J, Betriu A, et al. Management of acute myocardial infarction in patients presenting with persistent ST-segment elevation: the task force on the management of ST-segment elevation acute myocardial infarction of the European Society of Cardiology. Eur Heart J. 2008;29:2909–45.
5. Task Force for Diagnosis and Treatment of Non-ST-Segment Elevation Acute Coronary Syndromes of European Society of Cardiology, Bassand JP, Hamm CW, et al. Guidelines for the diagnosis and treatment of non-ST-segment elevation acute coronary syndromes. Eur Heart J. 2007;28:1598–660.
6. Walker DM, West NE, Ray SG, British Cardiovascular Society Working Group on Acute Cardiac Care. From coronary care unit to acute cardiac care unit: the evolving role of specialist cardiac care. Heart. 2012;98:350–2.
7. Hasin Y, Danchin N, Filippatos GS, et al. Recommendations for the structure, organization, and operation of intensive cardiac care units. Eur Heart J. 2005;26:1676–82.

8. Valle Tudela V, Alonso Garcia A, Aros Borau F, et al. Guidelines of the Spanish Society of Cardiology on requirements and equipment of the coronary care unit. Rev Esp Cardiol. 2001;54:617–23.
9. Di Chiara A, Chiarella F, Savonitto S, et al. BLITZ Investigators. Epidemiology of acute myocardial infarction in the Italian CCU network: the BLITZ study. Eur Heart J. 2003;24:1616–29.
10. Di Chiara A, Fresco C, Savonitto S, et al. On behalf of BLITZ-2 Investigators. Epidemiology of non-ST elevation acute coronary syndromes in the Italian cardiology network: the BLITZ-2 study. Eur Heart J. 2006;27:393–405.
11. Hasdai D, Behar S, Wallentin L, et al. A prospective survey of the characteristics, treatments and outcomes of patients with acute coronary syndromes in Europe and the Mediterranean basin; the Euro Heart Survey of Acute Coronary Syndromes (Euro Heart Survey ACS). Eur Heart J. 2002;23:1190–201.
12. Mandelzweig L, Battler A, Boyko V, et al. The second Euro Heart Survey on acute coronary syndromes: characteristics, treatment, and outcome of patients with ACS in Europe and the Mediterranean Basin in 2004. Eur Heart J. 2006;27:2285–93.
13. Lichtman JH, Spertus JA, Reid KJ, et al. Acute noncardiac conditions and in-hospital mortality in patients with acute myocardial infarction. Circulation. 2007;116:1925–30.
14. Granger CB, Goldberg RJ, Dabbous O, et al. Predictors of hospital mortality in the global registry of acute coronary events. Arch Intern Med. 2003;163:2345–53.
15. Valente S, Lazzeri C, Sori A, et al. The recent evolution of coronary care units into intensive cardiac care units: the experience of a tertiary center in Florence. J Cardiovasc Med. 2007;8:181–7.
16. Quinn T, Weston C, Birkhead J, et al. On behalf of the MINAP Steering Group. Redefining the coronary care unit: an observational study of patients admitted to hospital in England and Wales in 2003. Q J Med. 2005;98:797–802.
17. Katz JN, Turer AT, Becker RC. Cardiology and the critical care crisis: a perspective. J Am Coll Cardiol. 2007;49:1279–82.
18. Ferdinande P. Recommendations on minimal requirements for intensive care departments. Members of the task force of the European Society of Intensive Care Medicine. Intensive Care Med. 1997;23:226–32.
19. Casella G, Di Pasquale G. Competenza clinica del cardiologo dell'unità di terapia intensiva cardiologica [Clinical competence of the cardiologists working in coronary care units]. G Ital Cardiol. 2007;8(Suppl 1):16S–24S.
20. Bonnefoy-Cudraz E, Bueno H, Casella G, et al. Editor's choice—acute cardiovascular care association position paper on intensive cardiovascular care units: an update on their definition, structure, organisation and function. Eur Heart J Acute Cardiovasc Care. 2018;7:80–95.
21. Haupt MT, Bekes CE, Brilli RJ, et al. Guidelines on critical care services and personnel: recommendations based on a system of categorization of three levels of care. Crit Care Med. 2003;31:2677–83.
22. Schwab W, Frankel HL, Rotondo MF, et al. The impact of true partnership between a university Level I trauma center and a community Level II trauma center on patient transfer practices. J Trauma. 1998;44:815–9.
23. DiRusso S, Holly C, Kamath R, et al. Preparation and achievement of American College of Surgeons level I trauma verification raises hospital performance and improves patient outcome. J Trauma. 2001;51:294–9.
24. Na SJ, Chung CR, Jeon K, et al. Association between presence of a cardiac intensivist and mortality in an adult cardiac care unit. J Am Coll Cardiol. 2016;68:2637–48.
25. Morrow DA, Fang JC, Fintel DJ, et al. Evolution of critical care cardiology: transformation of the cardiovascular intensive care unit and the emerging need for new medical staffing and training models: a scientific statement from the American Heart Association. Circulation. 2012;126:1408–28.

26. Tubaro M, Vranckx P, Price S, et al. The ESC textbook of intensive and acute cardiovascular care. 2nd ed. London: Oxford University Press; 2015. p. 5–12.
27. Swetz KM, Mansel JK. Ethical issues and palliative care in the cardiovascular intensive care unit. Cardiol Clin. 2013;31:657–68.
28. Naib T, Lahewala S, Arora S, Gidwani U. Palliative care in the cardiac intensive care unit. Am J Cardiol. 2015;115:687–90.
29. Kappetein AP, Windecker S. The heart team in acute cardiovascular care. In: Tubaro M, Vranckx P, Price S, et al., editors. The ESC textbook of intensive and acute cardiovascular care. 2nd ed. London: Oxford University Press; 2015. p. 87–90.
30. Casella G, Cassin M, Chiarella F, et al. Epidemiology and patterns of care of patients admitted to Italian intensive cardiac care units: the BLITZ-3 registry. J Cardiovasc Med. 2010;11:450–61.
31. Visconti LO, Scorcu G, Cassin M, et al. Distribution and appropriateness of hospital admissions, resource utilization in the Italian intensive cardiac care units. The BLITZ-3 study. G Ital Cardiol (Rome). 2011;12(1):23–30.
32. Roubille F, Mercier G, Delmas C, et al. Description of acute cardiac care in 2014: a French nation-wide database on 277,845 admissions in 270 CICUs. Int J Cardiol. 2017;240:433–7.
33. Watson RA, Bohula EA, Gilliland TC, Sanchez PA, Berg DD, Morrow DA. Editor's choice - prospective registry of cardiac critical illness in a modern tertiary care cardiac intensive care unit. Eur Heart J Acute Cardiovasc Care. 2019;8(8):755–61.
34. Bohula EA, Katz JN, van Diepen S, et al. Demographics, care patterns, and outcomes of patients admitted to cardiac intensive care units: the critical care cardiology trials network prospective North American multicenter registry of cardiac critical illness. JAMA Cardiol. 2019;4(9):928–35.
35. Goldfarb M, van Diepen S, Liszkowski M, Jentzer JC, Pedraza I, Cercek B. Noncardiovascular disease and critical care delivery in a contemporary cardiac and medical intensive care unit. J Intensive Care Med. 2019;34(7):537–43.
36. Jentzer JC, van Diepen S, Barsness GW, et al. Changes in comorbidities, diagnoses, therapies and outcomes in a contemporary cardiac intensive care unit population. Am Heart J. 2019;215:12–9.
37. Bennett CE, Wright RS, Jentzer J, et al. Severity of illness assessment with application of the APACHE IV predicted mortality and outcome trends analysis in an academic cardiac intensive care unit. J Crit Care. 2019;50:242–6.
38. Holland EM, Moss TJ. Acute noncardiovascular illness in the cardiac intensive care unit. J Am Coll Cardiol. 2017;69(16):1999–2007.
39. Jentzer JC, Bennett C, Wiley BM, et al. Predictive value of the sequential organ failure assessment score for mortality in a contemporary cardiac intensive care unit population. J Am Heart Assoc. 2018;7(6):e008169.
40. Jentzer JC, Anavekar NS, Bennett C, et al. Derivation and validation of a novel cardiac intensive care unit admission risk score for mortality. J Am Heart Assoc. 2019;8(17):e013675.
41. Jentzer JC, Murphree DH, Wiley B, et al. Comparison of mortality risk prediction among patients ≥70 versus <70 years of age in a cardiac intensive care unit. Am J Cardiol. 2018;122(10):1773–8.
42. Katz JN, Minder M, Olenchock B, et al. The genesis, maturation, and future of critical care cardiology. J Am Coll Cardiol. 2016;68(1):67–79.
43. Teno JM, Gozalo P, Trivedi AN, et al. Site of death, place of care, and health care transitions among US Medicare beneficiaries, 2000-2015. JAMA. 2018;320(3):264–71.
44. Sinha SS, Sjoding MW, Sukul D, et al. Changes in primary noncardiac diagnoses over time among elderly cardiac intensive care unit patients in the United States. Circ Cardiovasc Qual Outcomes. 2017;10(8):e003616.
45. Bagshaw SM, Stelfox HT, McDermid RC, et al. Association between frailty and short- and long-term outcomes among critically ill patients: a multicentre prospective cohort study. CMAJ. 2014;186(2):E95–E102.

46. Forman DE, Arena R, Boxer R, et al. Prioritizing functional capacity as a principal end point for therapies oriented to older adults with cardiovascular disease: a scientific statement for healthcare professionals from the American Heart Association. Circulation. 2017;135(16):e894–918.
47. Damluji AA, Forman DE, van Diepen S, et al. Older adults in the cardiac intensive care unit: factoring geriatric syndromes in the management, prognosis, and process of care: a scientific statement from the American Heart Association. Circulation. 2020;141(2):e6–e32.
48. Katz JN, Sinha SS, Alviar CL, et al. COVID-19 and disruptive modifications to cardiac critical care delivery: JACC review topic of the week. J Am Coll Cardiol. 2020;76(1):72–84.

The Intensive and Advanced Treatments in the Cardiac Intensive Care Units

Alice Sacco, Luca Villanova, and Fabrizio Oliva

2.1 Introduction

Improvements in modern medicine had a deep impact on cardiovascular diseases (CVD): in the past decades we experienced a dramatic reduction in age-adjusted mortality among patients with CVD in every age group [1]. This extension in life span is linked, mostly in patients suffering from heart failure (HF), with an increased rate of polypharmacy, comorbidities, and disabilities that frequently progress to frailty syndrome, a medical condition that increases vulnerability to any type of stressors and reduces physiological reserves [2]. As a consequence it is more likely for patients with CVD, than for patients with other medical conditions, including cancer, to die in the hospital or other nursing facilities [3–5] (Fig. 2.1). Due to this epidemiologic scenario, the mean age at intensive care unit (ICU) admission is growing over time but CVD remains the most common clinical condition requiring intensive care. The diagnosis causing ICU admission in older patients with CVD has changed with a reduction of acute ischemic syndromes and an increase in decompensated HF complicated by cardiogenic shock and multiorgan failure with a very poor prognosis [6] (Fig. 2.2). Mortality from CVD is generally associated with a lower rate of treatment withdrawal, in comparison with noncardiovascular causes, especially in ICU wards [7]. Particularly relevant ethical issues come up in these settings as far as it concerns to discontinuation of medical therapies (including inotropes and vasopressors) and life-sustaining treatments (mechanical ventilation or renal replacement therapies) or deactivation of devices such as LVADs and cardiac implantable electrical devices (CIEDs).

A. Sacco (✉) · L. Villanova · F. Oliva
Intensive Cardiac Care Unit and De Gasperis Cardio Center, ASST Grande Ospedale Metropolitano Niguarda, Milan, Italy
e-mail: alice.sacco@ospedaleniguarda.it; luca.villanova@ospedaleniguarda.it; fabrizio.oliva@ospedaleniguarda.it

M. Romanò (ed.), *Palliative Care in Cardiac Intensive Care Units*,
https://doi.org/10.1007/978-3-030-80112-0_2

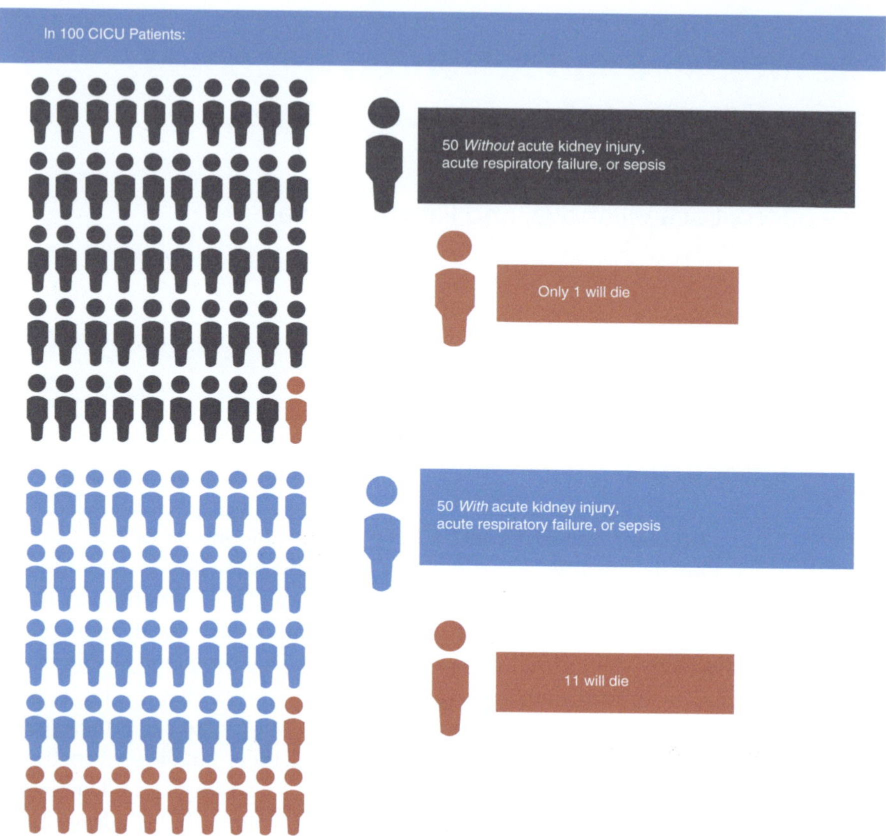

Fig. 2.1 Holland EM et al. J Am Coll Cardiol. 2017;69(16):1999–2007

Without the possibility to make a shared decision with the patients and their families and considering the difficult prognostication in terminally ill HF patients, clinicians are often struggling with initiating palliative care that is widely underused [8]. Consequently, intensivists and cardiologists are going, evermore, to be asked to face medical, ethical, and legal issues about end-of-life (EOL) and palliative care. Decisions about withholding and withdrawing life-sustaining treatments have to be made more frequently, without a detailed consensus from Scientific Societies and, often, an adequate legislative guidance. Older adults admitted to ICU should be reassessed shortly after the admission to weigh their level of care, even if age should not be considered the only criteria on decision-making [9, 10].

Palliative care should be seen no longer as a giving-up decision about treating CVD but as a supportive intervention for patients suffering from a chronic, critical, and life-limiting illness.

This approach is warranted by the epidemiological changes of the cardiac intensive care unit (CICU) that we have already highlighted: in particular in a review

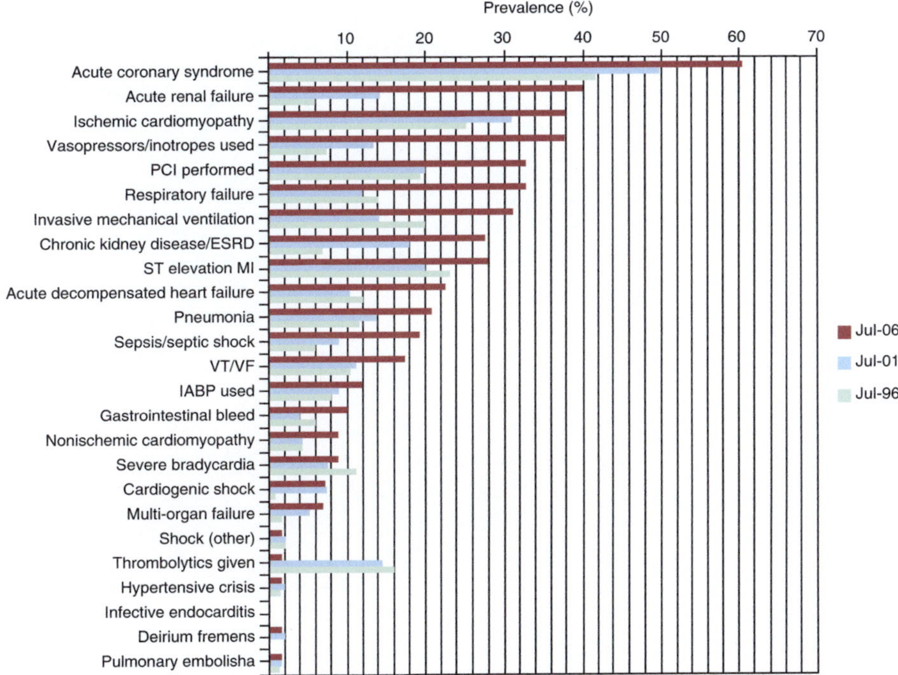

Fig. 2.2 Temporal trends of comorbidities and therapies (from Katz JN et al. Cardiology and the Critical Care Crisis A Perspective. J Am Coll Cardiol. 2007;49:1279–82)

by Katz [10] over a 17-year period from 1989 to 2006, rapid advances in innovation until the late 1990s led to a decrease in ST-segment elevation myocardial infarction (STEMI) mortality, but this was not true in patients with ischemic heart disease and advanced stages of HF.

As a consequence, there was an increased need of cardiologists with intensivist skills. In this context, it is essential to place the patient at the center at the time of admission, in order to adequately define the level and type of care/organ support needed.

Our coronary care unit, as it has occurred in the rest of Europe since the early 2000s, has been better characterized as cardiac intensive care unit (CICU), as a result of the change in the epidemiology of hospitalized patients, characterized by very complex clinical pictures: acute myocardial diseases complicated by cardiac arrests, advanced HF and cardiogenic shock, acute valvular pathology, prolonged arrhythmias, massive pulmonary embolism, iatrogenic complications of cardiac interventional procedures, cardiac patients admitted for noncardiac surgery, and congenital heart disease.

In January 2020, one month before the Covid-19 outbreak, the hospitalizations in our CICU were associated to the primary diagnosis showed in Fig. 2.3.

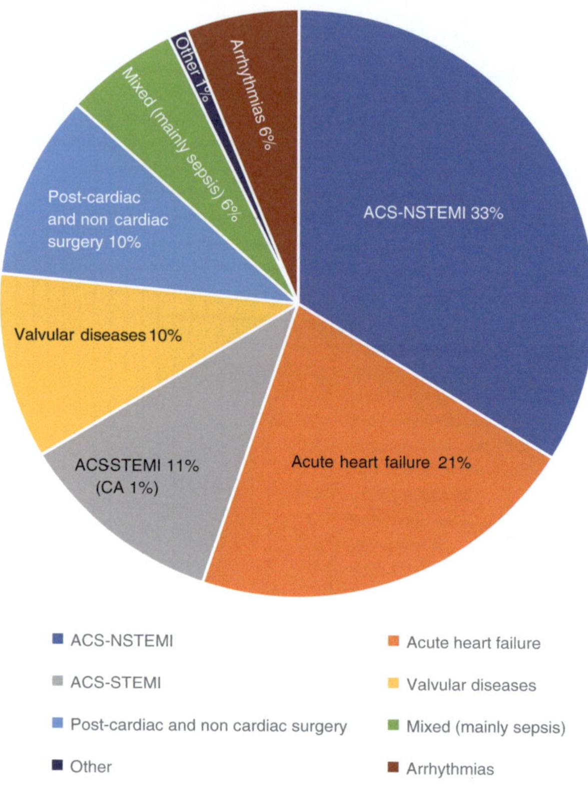

Fig. 2.3 Primary diagnosis in the month of January 2020 at CICU De Gasperis. *ACS* Acute Coronary Syndrome, *STEMI* ST Elevation Myocardial Infarction, *NSTEMI* Non ST Elevation Myocardial Infarction, *CA* Cardiac Arrest

2.2 Cardiac Arrest and Post-cardiac Arrest Syndrome

Cardiac arrest is the cause of approximately 500,000 deaths each year in Europe and the United States [1, 11]. Even if the majority of deaths occurs during the initial resuscitation maneuvers, a significant proportion happens during the post-resuscitation phase, mostly due to a combination of organ ischemia, reperfusion damage, and persisting pathophysiological processes that induces cardiac arrest (post-cardiac arrest syndrome). The impact of the post-cardiac arrest syndrome is more severe on the brain tissue that is particularly oxygen sensitive [12]. Neuronal injury is then exacerbated by loss of membrane resting potential, calcium-penetrating cells, and neurotransmitter release due to hypoxia [13]. After the restoration of blood flow circulation, reperfusion damage, stimulating inflammation, and release of oxygen free radicals cause a further direct damage to brain cells [14].

Targeted temperature management (TTM) has the purpose to diminish ischemia and reperfusion brain damage, lowering body temperature. Two clinical trials have demonstrated that TTM can reduce neurological dysfunction [15, 16], but only one of these proved TTM reduces mortality in patients with out-of-hospital cardiac arrest due to ventricular fibrillation [16]. In these studies patients were brought to a body temperature of 32–34 °C and hypothermia was prolonged for 12–24 h. TTM has been demonstrated to be effective in reducing neurological damage and improving survival also in case of non-shockable rhythms [17]. These data prompted TTM to be recommended by Scientific Societies guidelines in patients with out-of-hospital cardiac arrest due to ventricular fibrillation or pulseless ventricular tachycardia [18], despite the remaining doubts about the target temperature to achieve, timing, methods, and duration of this treatment.

In our CICU we practice TTM using a system that brings circulating chilled water in pads directly adherent to the patients' skin, sometimes in combination with core-cooling intravenous catheters with cold saline. When desired temperature is obtained, it should be maintained for a period of 12–24 h. To prevent shivering and to bring comfort to the patients, it is necessary to use sedatives and paralytics which can be discontinued once normothermia is settled again. To avoid hyperthermia and rewarming damages, temperature should be raised slowly at 0.25–0.5 °C/h.

A cardiac etiology of out-of-hospital cardiac arrest, including both coronary artery disease (CAD) and myocardial diseases, is very common. Several retrospective studies and postmortem analysis showed that there is a high rate of obstructive CAD (intended as epicardial coronary stenosis >50%) in patients with out-of-hospital cardiac arrest but it does not provide a clear cause to the event, especially when a coronary thrombus or a plaque rupture is absent [19, 20]. It has never been demonstrated that emergency coronary angiography and consequent percutaneous coronary intervention (PCI) have a clear benefit in patients with cardiac arrest, except for patients with ST-segment elevation or new left bundle branch block (LBBB) at the time of return of spontaneous circulation (ROSC). Indeed, patients with out-of-hospital cardiac arrest are often excluded from clinical trials evaluating the role of revascularization in acute settings; data are only available from observational studies and registries. The most recent meta-analysis including 15 observational studies in patients with cardiac arrest without ST-segment elevation or new onset of LBBB demonstrated an improved survival and lower neurological damages in the angiography group compared with delayed or no angiography [21]. Due to these data, cardiological Scientific Societies recommend to plan a coronary angiography in patients without ST-segment elevation myocardial infarction (STEMI) if there is a high suspicion of cardiac cause (chest pain, history of CAD, not clear electrocardiography results) and in the absence of other more favorable causes that can lead to the cardiac arrest [22, 23]. The Cardiac Arrest Hospital Prognosis (CAHP) score is a predictive tool to identify patients that will present poor neurological recovery after cardiac arrest at the ICU discharge [24]. A study sub-analysis showed that an early invasive strategy could be more effective in patients with lower predicted risk of brain damage, demonstrating that neurological, not cardiac, causes are linked with death in patients with most devastating forms of cardiac arrest [25]. In this scenario, the choice of an early coronary angiography strategy in patients with out-of-hospital cardiac arrest remains based on the clinical likelihood of obstructive CAD, futility of the intervention (extensive neurological damage, late resuscitation interventions), and hemodynamic instability.

Along with hypothermia and coronary angiography, patients with cardiac arrest need intensive monitoring and treatments. Due to the lack of clinical trials, intensive care measures are often guided by center-based experience and pathophysiology assumptions.

Hemodynamic support should be titrated on clinical features: vasopressors, fluids, inotropes, and mechanical circulatory support devices are used, upon clinician's judgement, to avoid arterial hypotension and worse outcome, especially in patients with myocardial dysfunction. 10–15% of patients after resuscitation from cardiac arrest suffer from seizures which are challenging to diagnose when sedatives and paralytics are used. Electroencephalographic (EEG) monitoring is mandatory, notably in patients treated with TTM, and an aggressive therapy of the first episode of seizures is advised but seizure prophylaxis is not recommended [26, 27]. Hyperglycemia is common in postarrest syndrome and can bring worsening of brain damage: glucose levels above 180 mg/dL should be treated with insulin, ideally with continuous infusion [28, 29]. Finally, accurate control of gas exchanges, electrolytes, and infection is recommended, in addition to appropriate diagnostic tests to find out and treat the cardiac arrest etiology.

The majority of patients with cardiac arrest do not die directly from hypoxic-ischemic brain injury but from withdrawal of life-sustaining treatments (WDLST) after a poor neurologic prognostication [30, 31]. As a consequence, a good prognostication process is mandatory to avoid premature WDLST: since none of the neurological predictors has 100% specificity, present guidelines recommend the use of a combination of tools such as clinical examination, serum biomarkers, neuroimaging, and electrophysiological tests (electroencephalogram and short-latency somatosensory evoked potentials) [32, 33].

Clinical neurological examination continues to be the milestone of prognostication after cardiac arrest: neuro-prognostication, starting from clinical examination, should be considered in every patient who is still unconscious and unresponsive to pain (Glasgow Coma Scale 2 or less), after 48–72 h of ROSC. Naturally, clinical tests for prognostication are vitiated by body temperature and use of paralytics and sedatives, confounders that should be ruled out every time starting neuro-prognostication.

Electroencephalogram (EEG) is one of the most used predictors but there is no homogenous classification of the different patterns: the Scientific Societies state that malignant results (status epilepticus or burst suppression without sedation and after rewarming) should be inserted in a multimodality analysis [32]. Recent evidences demonstrate that EEG can be an important neuro-prognostication tool even when it is recorded within 24 h after the cardiac arrest, despite low sensitivity [34]. As cited before, EEG is also useful to identify seizures that can worsen neurological damage with secondary injury. Absence of bilateral short-latency somatosensory evoked potentials (SSEP) at 72 h from cardiac arrest is one of the most potent neurological predictors, even if sensitivity is low [35]. Many patients with poor neurological outcome present bilateral SSEP but with low amplitude that should be considered as important as the complete absence of potentials in a multimodality stratification [36]. SSEP are advanced over EEG because they are less affected by sedative use but they are sensitive to body temperature and electric interferences [37].

Neuron-specific enolase (NSE) is a protein released by damaged neuronal cells and its blood values correlate with the extension of brain damage after cardiac arrest [38]. NSE concentration, compared with clinical examination and electrophysiology tests, is not affected by sedatives and paralytics and, as a biomarker, is an objective data, preventing clinician bias. On the contrary, as a continuous variable, NSE measurement does not have a clear threshold to identify patients with poor neurological outcome. In a large study on patients after cardiac arrest, NSE values with lower rate of false positives were 61, 46, and 35 ng/mL at 24, 48, and 72 h from ROSC [39]. Current guidelines recommend NSE measurement at different times (24, 48, and 72 h) to obtain more reproducible data [40]. NSE sampling should be used carefully because this biomarker can also be released by hemolysis, small-cell carcinoma, and neuroendocrine tumors.

Hypoxic-ischemic brain injury after cardiac arrest is documented by CT with cerebral edema that comes out as an attenuation of the gray matter and white matter interface measured by gray-white ratio (GWR). There is no consensus about timing for obtaining CT images but in the largest part of the studies CT is performed within 24 h with increased sensitivity on neurological outcome between 72 h and 7 days [41, 42]. MRI can show brain damage as hyperintense areas in diffusion-weighted images. MRI appears to be very accurate in predicting poor neurological outcome in postarrest syndrome but quantitative assessment is very heterogeneous. The Scientific Societies guidelines promote MRI use from 2 to 5 days after ROSC, even if recent studies show that it can be useful earlier, at 3 h [43, 44]. Due to lack of standardization in quantitative analysis and few scientific evidences, neuroimaging methods should be used in combination with the other predictors of neurological outcome to assure a good prognostication and prevent premature WDLST.

A multimodality prognostication algorithm should be used: firstly after rewarming patients from TTM, clinicians must exclude confounders, especially residual sedation. At 72 h, if pupillary light or corneal reflex is absent or SSEP waves are bilaterally absent or with low amplitude, poor neurological outcome is already very likely (false-positive rate <5%) and WDLST can be started. When at least one of these predictors is absent, patients should be re-evaluated after 24 h. At that time a poor neurological outcome is likely if two or more of the following tests are documented: status myoclonus within 48 h from ROSC, high NSE levels, malignant patterns at EEG, and diffuse anoxic injury at neuroimaging (TC or MRI). If these tests result to be inconclusive, WDLST should be avoided and patients re-evaluated on the basis of clinical evolution [32].

2.3   Advanced Heart Failure and End-Stage Heart Failure

Heart failure (HF) is a chronic illness characterized by a median survival of 2.1 years, a progressive decline in functional status, and a gradual increased severity of symptoms [45].

The goals of the treatment are:

- Hemodynamic improvement/stabilization (reduction of ventricular filling pressures, afterload and wall stress, improvement of cardiac contractility and coronary perfusion)
- Symptom control
- Improvement of organ function (oxygenation, renal and hepatic function)
- Improvement of prognosis

The severity of the clinical presentation and the pathophysiological profile, as well as the presence or absence of factors that have precipitated the decompensation and are susceptible to specific treatment, will guide the therapeutic management.

Diuretics are the cornerstone of acute heart failure (AHF) therapy. They are essential drugs to solve the picture of water overload and therefore they are used in the presence of signs/symptoms of pulmonary/peripheral congestion; radiological, bio-humoral, or blood gas data suggesting stasis; and high right and/or left ventricular filling pressures. Loop diuretics are the first-line drugs, usually administered intravenously in the first days of treatment. Different treatment regimens (refracted boluses vs. continuous infusion) have been compared in some clinical trials without, however, significant differences in the primary endpoints (improvement in symptoms and increased diuresis) [46].

The use of thiazide diuretics in combination finds its rationale in enhancing the pharmacological effect in patients in whom adequate diuresis is not obtained with loop diuretics. Ultrafiltration should be considered in patients resistant to diuretic therapy.

Vasodilator drugs are indicated in patients with signs of congestion and normal or high- or low-dose systemic blood pressure in the pictures of peripheral hypoperfusion associated with inotropic therapy. The most used drug is sodium nitroprusside (SNP) which leads to a reduction in systemic and pulmonary vascular resistances, with a consequent reduction of ventricular filling pressures and degree of mitral insufficiency, which results in an increased antegrade flow.

To reduce the risk of arterial hypotension, it should be titrated gradually starting from doses of 0.2 micrograms/kg/min up to a maximum tolerated dose, preferably by means of intra-arterial blood pressure monitoring. Prolonged use of the SNP may be associated with the toxicity of its plasma metabolite, the thiocyanide, which therefore must be monitored every 7–10 days, especially in patients with renal and/ or hepatic insufficiency.

Levosimendan has "mixed" characteristics, being an inodilator drug, differentiating itself for its unique pharmacodynamic and pharmacokinetic characteristics and for the greater availability of controlled clinical studies that have evaluated its efficacy and safety in patients with AHF. Thanks to its mechanism of action, it is effective in improving hemodynamic parameters and symptoms by promoting the normalization of ventricular-arterial coupling, and its use in patients with AHF is associated with better short- and medium-term survival [47].

Vasopressors, drugs with prominent peripheral arterial vasoconstrictive action such as norepinephrine, are administered to raise blood pressure and redistribute cardiac output from the periphery to vital organs. However, this is at the expense of an increase in left ventricular afterload. Their use should be limited to patients with persistent hypoperfusion despite adequate cardiac filling pressures.

2.4 Cardiogenic Shock (CS) and Low-Output Syndrome

Proper management of the patient in shock depends on the underlying cause. However, whatever the condition that leads to the picture of dysoxia, timely recourse to ventricular unloading with consequent improvement in peripheral perfusion and

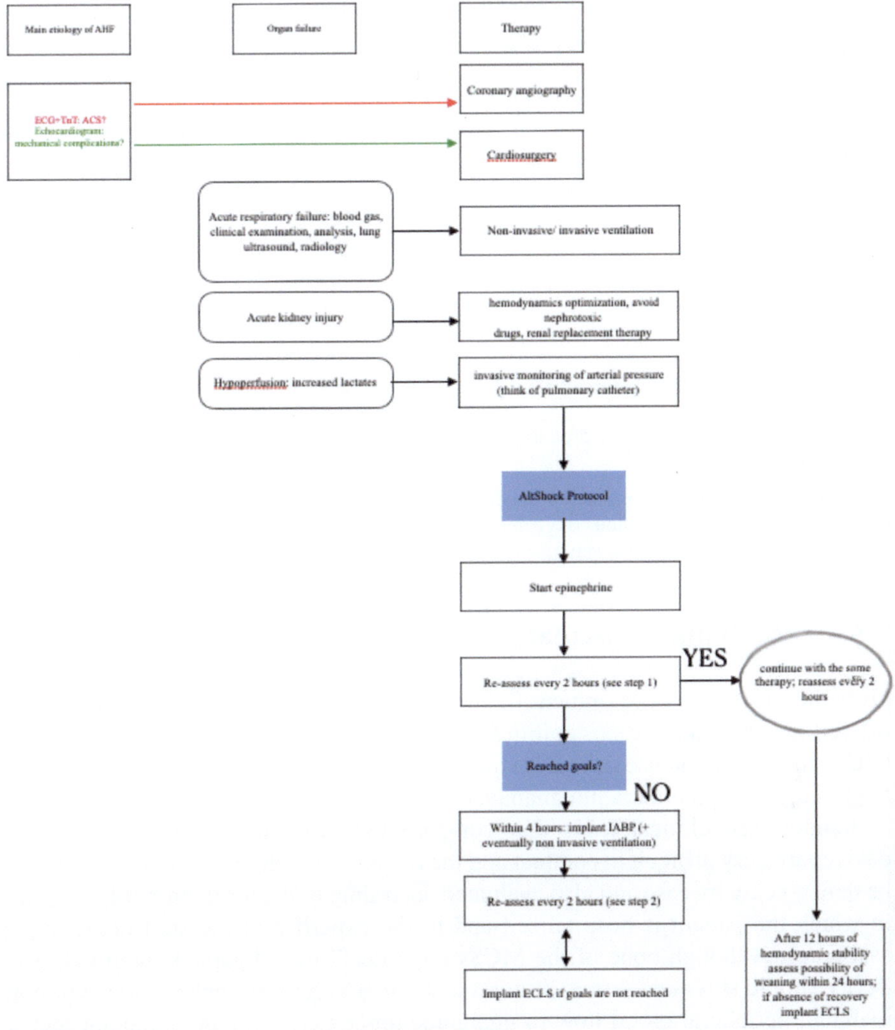

Fig. 2.4 Flowchart for the management of patients with low-output syndrome (modified from [49])

decrease in cardiac filling pressures is a fundamental tool to avoid irreversible organ damage and to improve the outcome [48].

In consideration of the high mortality related to slow-flow syndrome/CS, protocols/operative flowcharts are paramount to an early identification of this setting, in order to provide a quick, progressive therapeutic approach.

With this purpose, a protocol for the management of patients with low-output syndrome/CS has been developed in our department [49] (see Fig. 2.4; Table 2.1).

Table 2.1 Targets to reach at each step of the flowchart (modified from [49])

1st step: goal reached if at least 6/9 of the following If not: intensification of treatment with IABP and/or MV	*2nd step: goal reached if at least 5/8 of the following* If not: intensification of treatment with ECMO
Heart rate between 60 and 130 bpm	Heart rate between 60 and 130 bpm
Mean arterial pressure >65 mmHg	Mean arterial pressure >65 mmHg
$SVO_2 > 60\%$	$SVO_2 > 60\%$
$PaO_2 > 60$	$PaO_2 > 60$
Trend in serum lactate decrease	Lactates decrease $\geq 25\%$ with respect to V3
Respiratory rate <30/min	Wedge pressure <18 or E/E′ < 14
Diuresis >0.5 mL/kg/h	Diuresis >0.5 mL/kg/h
Epinephrine dose <0.07 mcg/kg/min	Epinephrine dose <0.12 mcg/kg/min without upgrade of other inotropes/vasopressors
Reduction of at least 20% compared to admission CVP	

IABP intra-aortic balloon pump, *MV* mechanical ventilation, *ECMO* extracorporeal membrane oxygenation, *SVO₂* mixed venous oxygen saturation measurements, *PaO₂* oxygen partial pressure, *V3* visit 3 (at 4 h), *CVP* central venous pressure, *Bpm* beats per minute

2.5 Mechanical Circulatory Supports (MCSs)

Over the years, the development of mechanical circulatory supports (MCSs) has offered new therapeutic possibilities to patients in cardiogenic shock assisted in CICU, though an intense debate is still active on the appropriate use of each device, the timing of implantation, the management methods, and the impact on prognosis.

Randomized clinical trials that compare the different ventricular assistance devices are very difficult to conduct and the use of one with respect to the other must be defined case by case and also evaluated according to the availability of the center in which the patient is hospitalized and to the expertise of the staff dedicated to assistance. Although none of the MCSs are "ideal" for all patients with CS, each device should still meet certain requirements such as ease of implantation, ability to maintain peripheral blood flow to guarantee organ perfusion and potential regression of alterations produced by low flow rate, ability to download the left ventricle, low rate of complications related to the implant, and permanence of assistance.

The initial hemodynamic goal of a MCS is to reduce preload, afterload, and myocardial oxygen consumption, with different modalities and efficacy depending on the device used. The final aim is to ensure adequate tissue perfusion in the passage towards functional recovery (bridge to recovery) or to a long-term support device (bridge to bridge) up to heart transplant (bridge to transplant).

The guidelines of the American Heart Association (Class IIa, Level of Evidence C) and the International Society for Heart and Lung Transplantation (Class 1C, Level of Evidence C) both recommend the placement of a "temporary" MCS in the INTERMACS 1 patient with multiorgan damage to allow adequate neurological evaluation and clinical laboratory optimization to evaluate indications for long-term MCS implantation and/or cardiac transplantation [50, 51].

- The intra-aortic balloon pump (IABP) is a device used since the 1960s, consisting of a balloon positioned inside the descending thoracic aorta and characterized by a rhythmic inflation/deflation synchronized with the cardiac cycle. It improves the systemic perfusion of the splanchnic organs, reducing the afterload in temporal correspondence with the ventricular systole, synchronous to the deflating phase of the balloon itself, and at the same time improving the coronary perfusion in diastole, synchronous to the inflated balloon. The increase in cardiac output is modest (about 0.5–1 L/min). There are absolute contraindications that preclude the use of IABP, such as the presence of aortic dissection, severe aortic insufficiency, and aortic intravascular stents. Among the relative contraindications there are severe peripheral vasculopathies, concomitant abdominal aortic aneurysm, significant thrombocytopenia, and severe sepsis. Scientific evidence shows the role of IABP in cardiogenic shock which is very controversial. In October 2012, Thiele et al. published the results of the IABP-SHOCK II trial [52].

  This is a prospective, multicenter, open-label study that randomized 600 patients with acute myocardial infarction complicated by cardiogenic shock to device implantation (IABP group, $n = 301$) or to treatment without IABP (control group, $n = 299$). There were no significant differences in study groups with respect to mortality at 30 days (primary endpoint: 39.7% in the IABP group versus 41.3% in the optimal medical therapy group, relative risk [RR] 0.96, 95% concomitance interval (CI), 0.79–1.17, $P = 0.69$) neither the time to hemodynamic stabilization, nor the time spent in the ICU, serum lactate levels, dose and duration of inotropic therapies, renal function, and adverse events. As a result of these studies, the 2016 ESC guidelines downgraded IABP to Class III with level of evidence B for the "routine" treatment of cardiogenic shock during acute myocardial infarction (AMI) [53]. Despite this, the "real-world" data reveals that to date the IABP remains the temporary support device to the frontline circle in these patients, given the wide availability and ease of implantation. Moreover, the negative or neutral results of the use of IABP in cardiogenic shock during AMI that emerged from the IABP-SHOCK II study cannot be generalized to other conditions of cardiogenic shock not related to acute coronary syndrome.

- The Impella is a family of mechanical assistance devices consisting of a microaxial pump placed via a retrograde approach across the aortic valve using a femoral arterial access; the distal end of the catheter pumps blood from the left ventricle into the ascending aorta and systemic circulation, thus ensuring the emptying of the left ventricular cavity. Impella 2.5 and Impella CP are positioned percutaneously, generally under fluoroscopic guidance, through the femoral or axillary artery, and, respectively, guarantee 2.5 L/min and 3.7–4 L/min of estimated flow. Impella 5.0 requires surgical isolation of the artery for catheter placement, which guarantees up to 5 L/min of estimated flow. The hemodynamic effect is given by the venting of the left ventricle with a reduction in stroke work and myocardial oxygen consumption. The main limitations are related to the high rotation speed of the axial pump with the risk of hemolysis and the incidence of femoral bleeding and ischemia of the lower limb due to the femoral insertion of the cannula. Its placement is contraindicated in patients with severe aortic valve insufficiency, mechanical aortic valve prosthesis, and severe peripheral vasculopathy. Also to the same "family" belongs the Impella RD, a support device for the right ventricle, consisting of a catheter (22 Fr) positioned in the femoral vein up to the pulmonary valve. The device draws blood from the inferior vena cava and pumps it into the pulmonary artery, ensuring an estimated maximum flow of 4 L/min, the effect of which consists of a reduction in central venous pressure and an increase in cardiac index.

- TandemHeart consists of a system equipped with a continuous centrifugal pump that guarantees hemodynamic support of about 6 L/min. A cannula is inserted via femoral vein access and pushed into the left atrium through transseptal puncture; oxygenated blood is aspirated from the left atrium and pushed into the abdominal aorta or an iliac artery using a second cannula placed in the femoral artery. The hemodynamic advantage is undoubted compared to the IABP: there is a significant increase in cardiac output and mean arterial pressure and a decrease in pulmonary resistance, central venous pressure, and pulmonary artery pressure. Reducing biventricular filling pressures decreases myocardial workload and oxygen demand. Complications related to the TandemHeart implant are accidental left atrial perforation at the time of transseptal puncture, dissection of the common femoral artery, inguinal hematoma, bleeding at the site of cannula insertion, ischemia in the lower limb, sepsis, gastrointestinal bleeding, coagulopathy, need for transfusion, and stroke. The maximum duration of the implant is 2 weeks.

- Extracorporeal membrane oxygenation (ECMO) system consists of a system of inflow and outflow cannula, a centrifugal pump, and an oxygenating membrane, which replaces the heart and lung. The ECMO cannulas can be positioned percutaneously or with surgical isolation of the vessel used, to bedside, even though they are large cannulas. The most commonly used vessels are the femoral vein and artery; however also the subclavian artery and internal jugular vein can provide accesses for cannulation. An antegrade cannula is also placed in the femoral artery in order to ensure adequate limb perfusion. The ECMO provides total circulatory support (flow rate from 4.5 to 7 L/min). The hemodynamic result is a preload decrease without however causing decompression of the left ventricle; therefore, in order to reduce the afterload and oxygen consumption, a left ventricular "venting" device such as the IABP or the Impella can be positioned [53].

- ECMO has undisputed advantages such as high hemodynamic support, relative speed and ease of positioning, and presence of an oxygenation membrane capable of rapidly improving tissue oxygenation by bypassing the alveolar-capillary interface, compromised by the concomitant presence of CS and severe pulmonary congestion.

  However its use exposes the patient to many important possible complications mainly of ischemic and/or hemorrhagic type (ischemia of the lower limb, bleeding, endoventricular thrombosis, thromboembolism), renal damage, cerebrovascular and gastrointestinal adverse events, systemic inflammatory response syndrome (SIRS), or ECMO technical dysfunction.

2.6   Heart Replacement Therapies

Due to the limited therapeutic options for patients with end-stage heart failure, long-term MCS is continuously growing in use: between 2006 and 2010 in the United States 2680 adults received a left ventricular assist device (LVAD). 82% were listed for orthotopic heart transplant at the time of implant (bridge to transplant) or as bridge to candidacy, and the rest were as destination therapy. 87% of patients implanted as bridge to transplant were still alive or have been transplanted at 12-month follow-up, compared with 67% of those implanted as destination therapy [54]. Factors influencing the duration of long-term MCS and survival were timing of implant, patient's age, and medical comorbidities. Although quality of life, functional status (longer distances at the 6-min walking test), and NYHA functional class improve after long-term MCS implantation, related complications can hardly affect patients' and their caregivers' quality of life. Furthermore, because of the longevity gained by long-term MCS implantation, patients can show progression of cardiovascular or non-cardiovascular disease, experiencing end of life along with the device still on. The use of long-term MCS definitely alters the natural process of end-stage HF. Patients with long-term MCS devices can potentially die in the early postsurgical period, after an acute event in the months or years after implantation or after terminal decline. The most common and deadly complications related to long-term MCS are stroke, progressive HF, bleedings, infections, and multiorgan failure [55]. One of the most concerning complications is disabling stroke that has a very high prevalence in patients implanted with long-term MSC (between 3 and 12% in HeartMate II recipients [54]). Such events should be considered a trigger to reassess heart replacement therapy, changing the benefit/risk ratio, especially for patients with devices implanted as destination therapy. Palliative care should always be involved in the managing of patients with long-term MCS. At the beginning, when the device is considered for the first time, palliative care physicians can assist heart team in patient understanding of the purpose and the limitations of the device. They can further support in preparing the patient and his/her relatives and/or caregivers for life changes that are device related (battery changes, troubleshooting alarms, driveline site managing).

Clinical scenarios that can lead to LVAD deactivation are ruinous complication such as stroke, sepsis, and multiorgan failure; poor quality of life despite long-term MCS due to chronic infections, frequent hospitalizations, and denial of other life-sustaining treatments like hemodialysis; and advance of other comorbidities such as dementia and cancer [56, 57]. Long-term MCS deactivation frequently occurs in ICU, with simultaneous withdrawal of other life-sustaining treatments as renal replacement therapies, mechanical ventilation, and medical therapy [58]. The resolution about long-term MCS withdrawal should be collegial, engaging the patient, surrogate decision maker when the patient is incompetent, relatives, caregivers, and multidisciplinary clinical team members, including palliative care physicians. The deactivation process and its consequences should be clearly described and concerns from all the people involved should be addressed. Because the process often occurs in the hospital and mostly in the ICU, families and loved ones should be allowed to frequently visit the patient. Life span after long-term MCS deactivation can vary, from minutes to few days; this should be well outlined to relatives to prevent wrong reactions about time to death longer or shorter than expected [59]. Withdrawal of the other life-sustaining treatments should be pursued, reassuring patient and the family that patient comfort is granted. Each monitoring that is not focused on symptom control should be discontinued. Clinicians must be prepared to prevent and treat the prompt outbreak of signs of patient discomfort and symptoms such as dyspnea, labored respiration, and agitation. Due to low cardiac output state, comfort therapies such as opioids, benzodiazepines, and diuretics can have a retarded time to peak effect.

In the last decades, orthotopic cardiac transplantation turned out to be a crucial therapeutic option in patients with end-stage heart diseases, improving survival and quality of life. Survival rates after cardiac transplant are 88% for men and 86.2% for women at 1 year and 73.2% for men and 69% for women at 5 years [1]. Physical and emotional symptoms such as dyspnea, pain, and depression are often under-addressed in patients who are candidates to or who have received heart transplantation [60]. Patients waiting for transplant often experience multimodal distress also because of clinical uncertainty, long waiting periods, and anxiety about transplant success. In the pre-heart transplant period, palliative care interventions can improve quality of life and reduce anxiety with increasing satisfaction about continuity of care [60]. In the post-heart transplant period, even if quality of life improves along with reduction of symptom burden, patients can continue to feel pain from mild to severe degree [61, 62]. Patients struggle to return to normal life including work, personal relationships, and sexual life [63]. Almost 30% of patients after heart transplant complain of depression, resulting in less adequate compliance to complex therapies (immunosuppression) and invasive procedures at follow-up (myocardial biopsy and coronary angiography) and in more frequent hospitalizations. Palliative care can improve therapy adherence and quality of life, improving subjective aspects related to medical care after heart transplantation.

2.7 Cardiac Implanted Electronic Devices (CIEDs)

The number of cardiac implantable electronic device (CIED) procedures is constantly increasing worldwide, in primary or secondary prevention of sudden cardiac death (implantable cardioverter-defibrillator—ICD) or as a treatment of left ventricular dysfunction and left bundle branch block (cardiac resynchronization therapy—CRT, in selected cases associated with defibrillator—CRTD). Despite the great benefits deriving from CIED, issues are rising about the device management in patients at the end of life, when death is a result from either CVD deterioration or other end-stage chronic diseases.

The rationale for CIED deactivation, in particular ICDs and CRT-Ds, is to avoid unnecessary and painful, multiple shock delivered to a patient in the last weeks or hours before death. In a recent study, in a population of 100 patients 97 still had anti-tachycardia therapies activated in the last 24 h before death and 32% of these received at least one shock (10 patients received more than 10 shocks) in this short period of time at the end of life [64]. Deactivation of implantable electronic devices is often not recognized as one of the most important steps in the palliative care of patients suffering end-stage cardiovascular and non-cardiovascular diseases [65, 66]. Receiving ICD or CRT-D shocks not only is uncomfortable for patients in their last hours of life but can also badly affect family members and caregivers with significant pain and distress [64].

For details about this topic see Chap. 5.

2.8 Palliative Care in CICU

When the illness progresses to Stage D of the American College of Cardiology/ American Heart Association, i.e., end-stage heart failure, patients present poor quality of life, higher and more severe symptom burden, and a life span between 6 and 12 months [67]. In these last months of life, heart failure patients often face recurrent hospital admissions, medical procedures, and intensive care use, bringing in-hospital death.

However a recent study demonstrates that, in a period between 2003 and 2017, an increasing number of HF-related cardiovascular deaths are occurring in hospice facilities and at home (respectively 0.2–8.2% and 20.6–30.7%), with fewer deaths occurring in hospital.

Nevertheless cardiovascular-HF patients are still less likely to die in hospice facilities or at home than patients dying of cancer [68], even if the majority of patients express the will to die at home and to want less intensive care at end of life [69].

Scientific Societies guidelines emphasize that palliative care should be considered for patients with advanced heart failure and that it should be introduced in the early phases of the disease and increased over the disease progression [70, 71]. Lately, the prognostication model with the recognition of end of life as a trigger to begin palliative care in patients with heart failure has been reconsidered in a symptom-center model because of the prognostic uncertainty in CVD due to the poor utility of the present prognostic scores [72].

2.9 Palliative Inotrope Care

Several trials (REVIVE II, OPTIME CHF, and PROMISE [73–75]) have raised some concerns about the use of intravenous or oral inotropes in the setting of acute and chronic heart failure, showing a reduction in survival and a more elevated risk of cardiovascular events: survival at 6-month follow-up was less than 50%. However, these studies were conducted before current evidences about optimal medical therapy in heart failure patients, including neurohormonal agents, chronic resynchronization therapy (CRT), and implantable cardioverter-defibrillator (ICD). Furthermore, they do not include the use of inotropes as palliative care. More recent studies showed an improved survival maybe due to lower doses of inotropes and better HF clinical intervention management. A recent review about the use of inotropes in heart failure patients demonstrated an improvement in functional status (patients gained at least one class in the New York Heart Association—NYHA—classification), without any effect on survival [76]. The most common inotrope used was dobutamine (74.2% of studies), while dopamine was employed in 37.8%, levosimendan in 15.2%, and milrinone in 10.6% of studies. Inotropes were more often administered intermittently than continuously (50.0% vs. 31.8%, respectively). The indications to inotropes were palliative therapy in only 12% of studies, bridge to transplant in 17%, and unspecified in 51%. Scientific guidelines for HF affirm that continuous palliative inotropic therapy may be considered in patients with stage D heart failure who are not eligible for therapies upgraded with mechanical circulatory support or heart transplantation [70, 77]. However identifying which patient may benefit from palliative inotrope infusion can be challenging.

Clinical features that can be considered in the decision of starting palliative inotrope therapy include stage D heart failure with NYHA IV class symptoms that improve during the infusion and worsen at withdrawal. Most prevalent causes of impossible weaning from inotropes were end-organ hypoperfusion (22%), arterial hypotension (17%), and arterial hypotension with renal dysfunction (9%) [78]. Weaning attempts should be made on in-hospital basis and before declaring a patient inotrope dependent the HF team should consider other acute medical issues in a clinical scenario often burdened by comorbidities. Before starting with this advanced and clinical demanding therapy, other medications should be optimized, up-titrating opioids and diuretics. A comprehensive hemodynamic assessment should be made over symptoms, blood pressure, physical examination, and blood testing, to identify the most effective and the lowest dose to maintain hemodynamic stability and symptom improvement without exacerbation of arrhythmias. Patients suffering from aortic stenosis, pulmonary stenosis, and left ventricular outflow tract obstruction should be excluded. Uncontrolled and refractory arrythmias should be considered as a relative contraindication and, if possible, should be controlled and addressed during the in-hospital inotrope infusion. Severe renal dysfunction is a relative contraindication, especially when milrinone is considered as a palliative inotrope. Starting with palliative inotrope therapy should always follow the assessment of patient goals and values, family support, and psychological evaluation. The patient and his/her family must be aware that other advanced therapies have been excluded and they should be informed about risks, benefits, and possible death. Treatment withdrawal should always be considered an option when complication, ineffectiveness, or imminent death occurs. Inotrope therapy, both as bridge to heart replacement therapy or as palliative treatment, improves functional status and symptoms, although is not clear if it is a placebo effect [76, 78, 79].

The prevailing complications associated with palliative inotrope therapy are infections and arrhythmias with appropriate or inappropriate ICD shocks. Other complications can be tachyphylaxis, persistent heart failure symptoms, and myocardial ischemia but they are rare. The pooled incidence of ICD shocks in patients with continuous inotrope therapy is 2.4% per months of follow-up [76]. In a recent study, 17% of patients with end-stage heart failure treated with palliative inotropes had one or more ICD shocks, 18% of which were inappropriate [79]. Low ejection fraction, history of arrhythmic pattern, and chronic use of ACE inhibitors are strong predictors of ICD shocks during the treatment, in contrast with inotrope dose that does not correlate [79]. Central line complications have a cumulative rate of 3.6% per months of follow-up and the more frequently reported are infection as bacteremia with only 10% limited locally [76, 80]. Other complications linked to central line use in palliative inotrope therapy are occlusion due to thrombosis, endocarditis, and need for dedicated caregiver.

In the palliative care, currently inotropes used are milrinone, dobutamine, dopamine, and levosimendan. Hashim et al. reported a longer median survival in patients treated with milrinone compared with dobutamine but inotrope choice was not randomized (85% of the population was treated with milrinone) [81]. In contrast, Gorodeski et al. demonstrated no statistical difference in adjusted mortality after a median follow-up of 130 days in patients treated with milrinone or dobutamine [82]. The inodilator levosimendan may be advantageous in the palliative care or end-of-life settings, not least because of its sustained duration of action, ascribed to a long-acting metabolite, and is not associated with increased mortality [83]. Consequently, because of the lack of clear evidences, the inotrope choice should be individualized on the patient characteristics and on the heart failure team expertise.

Regular follow-up should be dictated by the clinical setting and by the treatment target decided with patient and his/her family. The most relevant monitoring should be about symptoms and quality of life, along with serum electrolytes and renal function. Rapid changes in weight without exacerbation of heart failure symptoms can be an alert of worsening clinical status.

Tachyphylaxis can reduce inotrope effectiveness over time and a dose titration should be considered to maintain symptom control [84].

Inotrope withdrawal should be performed slowly and conducted following a protocol shared with the patient, his/her family, and his/her caregivers. Withdrawal should be performed when inotropes are ineffective in improving patients' quality of life and symptom burden or when the patient is imminently dying. Infections should prompt hospital admission and antibiotic therapy, considering central line removal and reassessment of utility and feasibility of palliative inotrope therapy. When ICD shocks frequently occur, initiation of anti-arrhythmic drugs, inotrope dosage reduction to complete withdrawal, or deactivation of anti-tachycardia therapies should be considered, sharing the decision with the patient and with an electrophysiology expert. Once inotrope withdrawal is made, patients, especially those with low blood pressure and low cardiac output state, can die in minutes: symptoms that can occur in these moments should be anticipated and palliative medications such as opioids and diuretics should be administered in anticipation [85–87].

References

1. Virani SS, Alonso A, Benjamin EJ, et al. Heart disease and stroke statistics—2020 update: a report from the American Heart Association. Circulation. 2020;141(9):e139–596.
2. Yang Y, Lee LC. Dynamics and heterogeneity in the process of human frailty and aging: evidence from the U.S. older adult population. J Gerontol Ser B Psychol Sci Soc Sci. 2010;65B(2):246–55.
3. Weitzen S, Teno JM, Fennell M, Vincent MOR. Factors associated with site of death a national study of where people die. Med Care. 2003;41:323–35.
4. Cohen J, Houttekier D, Chambaere K, Bilsen J, Deliens L. The use of palliative care services associated with better dying circumstances. Results from an epidemiological population-based study in the Brussels metropolitan region. J Pain Symptom Manag. 2011;42:839–51.
5. Van Der Plas AGM, Oosterveld-Vlug MG, Pasman HRW, Onwuteaka-Philipsen BD. Relating cause of death with place of care and healthcare costs in the last year of life for patients who died from cancer, chronic obstructive pulmonary disease, heart failure and dementia: a descriptive study using registry data. Palliat Med. 2017;31:338–45.
6. Sjoding MW, Prescott HC, Wunsch H, Iwashyna TJ, Cooke CR. Longitudinal changes in ICU admissions among elderly patients in the United States. Crit Care Med. 2016;44:1353–60.
7. Orban J-C, Walrave Y, Mongardon N, et al. Causes and characteristics of death in intensive care units. Anesthesiology. 2017;126:882–9.
8. Guidet B, De Lange DW, Christensen S, et al. Attitudes of physicians towards the care of critically ill elderly patients—a European survey. Acta Anaesthesiol Scand. 2018;62:207–19.
9. Sprung CL, Woodcock T, Sjokvist P, et al. Reasons, considerations, difficulties and documentation of end-of-life decisions in European intensive care units: The ETHICUS Study. Intensive Care Med. 2008;34:271–7.
10. Katz JN, Shah BR, Volz EM, et al. Evolution of the coronary care unit: clinical characteristics and temporal trends in healthcare delivery and outcomes. Crit Care Med. 2010;38:375–81.
11. Atwood C, Eisenberg MS, Herlitz J, Rea TD. Incidence of EMS-treated out-of-hospital cardiac arrest in Europe. Resuscitation. 2005;67:75–80.
12. Madl C, Holzer M. Brain function after resuscitation from cardiac arrest. Curr Opin Crit Care. 2004;10:213–7.
13. Hoesch RE, Koenig MA, Geocadin RG. Coma after global ischemic brain injury: pathophysiology and emerging therapies. Crit Care Clin. 2008;24:25–44.
14. Lee JM, Grabb MC, Zipfel GJ, Choi DW. Brain tissue responses to ischemia. J Clin Invest. 2000;106:723–31.
15. Bernard SA, Gray TW, Buist MD, et al. Treatment of comatose survivors of out-of-hospital cardiac arrest with induced hypothermia. N Engl J Med. 2002;346:557–63.
16. Hypothermia after Cardiac Arrest Study Group. Mild therapeutic hypothermia to improve the neurologic outcome after cardiac arrest. N Engl J Med. 2002;346:549–56.
17. Lascarrou J-B, Merdji H, Le Gouge A, et al. Targeted temperature management for cardiac arrest with nonshockable rhythm. N Engl J Med. 2019;381:2327–37.
18. Panchal AR, Bartos JA, Cabañas JG, et al. Part 3: Adult basic and advanced life support: 2020 American Heart Association Guidelines for cardiopulmonary resuscitation and emergency cardiovascular care. Circulation. 2020;142(16_suppl_2):S366–468.
19. Radsel P, Knafelj R, Kocjancic S, Noc M. Angiographic characteristics of coronary disease and postresuscitation electrocardiograms in patients with aborted cardiac arrest outside a hospital. Am J Cardiol. 2011;108:634–8.
20. Dumas F, Cariou A, Manzo-Silberman S, et al. Immediate percutaneous coronary intervention is associated with better survival after out-of-hospital cardiac arrest. Circ Cardiovasc Interv. 2010;3:200–7.
21. Camuglia AC, Randhawa VK, Lavi S, Walters DL. Cardiac catheterization is associated with superior outcomes for survivors of out of hospital cardiac arrest: review and meta-analysis. Resuscitation. 2014;85:1533–40.

22. Collet J-P, Thiele H, Barbato E, et al. ESC guidelines for the management of acute coronary syndromes in patients presenting without persistent ST-segment elevation. Eur Heart J. 2020;2020:ehaa575. https://doi.org/10.1093/eurheartj/ehaa575.
23. Noc M, Fajadet J, Lassen JF, et al. Invasive coronary treatment strategies for out-of-hospital cardiac arrest: a consensus statement from the European association for percutaneous cardiovascular interventions (EAPCI)/stent for life (SFL) groups. EuroIntervention. 2014;10:31–7.
24. Maupain C, Bougouin W, Lamhaut L, et al. The CAHP (Cardiac Arrest Hospital Prognosis) score: a tool for risk stratification after out-of-hospital cardiac arrest. Eur Heart J. 2016;37:3222–8.
25. Bougouin W, Dumas F, Karam N, et al. Should we perform an immediate coronary angiogram in all patients after cardiac arrest? Insights from a large French Registry. JACC Cardiovasc Interv. 2018;11:249–56.
26. Rittenberger JC, Popescu A, Brenner RP, Guyette FX, Callaway CW. Frequency and timing of nonconvulsive status epilepticus in comatose post-cardiac arrest subjects treated with hypothermia. Neurocrit Care. 2012;16:114–22.
27. Amorim E, Rittenberger JC, Baldwin ME, Callaway CW, Popescu A, Post Cardiac Arrest Service. Malignant EEG patterns in cardiac arrest patients treated with targeted temperature management who survive to hospital discharge. Resuscitation. 2015;90:127–32.
28. Beiser DG, Carr GE, Edelson DP, Peberdy MA, Hoek TLV. Derangements in blood glucose following initial resuscitation from in-hospital cardiac arrest: a report from the national registry of cardiopulmonary resuscitation. Resuscitation. 2009;80:624–30.
29. Jacobi J, Bircher N, Krinsley J, et al. Guidelines for the use of an insulin infusion for the management of hyperglycemia in critically ill patients. Crit Care Med. 2012;40:3251–76.
30. Dragancea I, Wise MP, Al-Subaie N, et al. Protocol-driven neurological prognostication and withdrawal of life-sustaining therapy after cardiac arrest and targeted temperature management. Resuscitation. 2017;117:50–7.
31. Mulder M, Gibbs HG, Smith SW, et al. Awakening and withdrawal of life-sustaining treatment in cardiac arrest survivors treated with therapeutic hypothermia. Crit Care Med. 2014;42:2493–9.
32. Sandroni C, Cariou A, Cavallaro F, et al. Prognostication in comatose survivors of cardiac arrest: an advisory statement from the European resuscitation council and the European society of intensive care medicine. Resuscitation. 2014;85:1779–89.
33. Nolan JP, Soar J, Cariou A, et al. European Resuscitation Council and European Society of Intensive Care Medicine 2015 guidelines for post-resuscitation care. Intensive Care Med. 2015;41:2039–56.
34. Sondag L, Ruijter BJ, Tjepkema-Cloostermans MC, et al. Early EEG for outcome prediction of postanoxic coma: prospective cohort study with cost-minimization analysis. Crit Care. 2017;21:111.
35. Solari D, Rossetti AO, Carteron L, et al. Early prediction of coma recovery after cardiac arrest with blinded pupillometry. Ann Neurol. 2017;81:804–10.
36. Endisch C, Storm C, Ploner CJ, Leithner C. Amplitudes of SSEP and outcome in cardiac arrest survivors: a prospective cohort study. Neurology. 2015;85:1752–60.
37. Bouwes A, Binnekade JM, Kuiper MA, et al. Prognosis of coma after therapeutic hypothermia: a prospective cohort study. Ann Neurol. 2012;71:206–12.
38. Cronberg T, Rundgren M, Westhall E, et al. Neuron-specific enolase correlates with other prognostic markers after cardiac arrest. Neurology. 2011;77:623–30.
39. Stammet P, Collignon O, Hassager C, et al. Neuron-specific enolase as a predictor of death or poor neurological outcome after out-of-hospital cardiac arrest and targeted temperature management at 33°C and 36°C. J Am Coll Cardiol. 2015;65:2104–14.
40. Wiberg S, Hassager C, Stammet P, et al. Single versus serial measurements of neuron-specific enolase and prediction of poor neurological outcome in persistently unconscious patients after out-of-hospital cardiac arrest—a TTM-trial substudy. PLoS One. 2017;12:e0168894. https://doi.org/10.1371/journal.pone.0168894.

41. Choi SP, Park HK, Park KN, et al. The density ratio of grey to white matter on computed tomography as an early predictor of vegetative state or death after cardiac arrest. Emerg Med J. 2008;25:666–9.
42. Lee BK, Kim WY, Shin J, et al. Prognostic value of gray matter to white matter ratio in hypoxic and non-hypoxic cardiac arrest with non-cardiac etiology. Am J Emerg Med. 2016;34:1583–8.
43. Park JS, Lee SW, Kim H, et al. Efficacy of diffusion-weighted magnetic resonance imaging performed before therapeutic hypothermia in predicting clinical outcome in comatose cardiopulmonary arrest survivors. Resuscitation. 2015;88:132–7.
44. Mlynash M, Campbell DM, Leproust EM, et al. Temporal and spatial profile of brain diffusion-weighted MRI after cardiac arrest. Stroke. 2010;41:1665–72.
45. Ko DT, Alter DA, Austin PC, et al. Life expectancy after an index hospitalization for patients with heart failure: a population-based study. Am Heart J. 2008;155:324–31.
46. Felker GM, Lee KL, Bull DA. Diuretic strategies in persons with acute decompensated heart failure. N Engl J Med. 2011;364:797–805.
47. Altenberger J, Gustafsson F, Harjola VP, et al. Levosimendan in acute and advanced heart failure: an appraisal of the clinical database and evaluation of its therapeutic applications. J Cardiovasc Pharmacol. 2018;71:129–36.
48. Viola G, Morici N, Sacco A, et al. Cardiogenic shock: old and new circulatory assist devices: the role of counter-pulsation. Eur Heart J Suppl. 2019;21:B59–60.
49. Morici N, Oliva F, Ajello S, et al. Management of cardiogenic shock in acute decompensated chronic heart failure: the ALTSHOCK phase II clinical trial. Am Heart J. 2018;204:196–201.
50. Cook JL, Colvin M, Francis GS, et al. Recommendations for the use of mechanical circulatory support: ambulatory and community patient care: a scientific statement from the American Heart Association. Circulation. 2017;135:e1145–58.
51. Feldman D, Pamboukian SV, Teuteberg JJ, et al. The 2013 International Society for heart and lung transplantation guidelines for mechanical circulatory support: executive summary. J Heart Lung Transplant. 2013;32:157–87.
52. Thiele H, Zeymer U, Neumann FJ, et al. Intra-aortic balloon counterpulsation in acute myocardial infarction complicated by cardiogenic shock (IABP-SHOCK II): final 12 month results of a randomised, open-label trial. Lancet. 2013;382:1638–45.
53. Soleimani B, Pae WE. Management of left ventricular distension during peripheral extracorporeal membrane oxygenation for cardiogenic shock. Perfus (United Kingdom). 2012;27:326–31.
54. Kirklin JK, Naftel DC, Pagani FD, et al. Seventh INTERMACS annual report: 15,000 patients and counting. J Hear Lung Transplant. 2015;34:1495–504.
55. Dunlay SM, Strand JJ, Wordingham SE, Stulak JM, Luckhardt AJ, Swetz KM. Dying with a left ventricular assist device as destination therapy. Circ Heart Fail. 2016;9:1–9.
56. Swetz KM, Ottenberg AL, Freeman MR, Mueller PS. Palliative care and end-of-life issues in patients treated with left ventricular assist devices as destination therapy. Curr Heart Fail Rep. 2011;8:212–8.
57. Verdoorn BP, Luckhardt AJ, Wordingham SE, Dunlay SM, Swetz KM. Palliative medicine and preparedness planning for patients receiving left ventricular assist device as destination therapy—challenges to measuring impact and change in institutional culture. J Pain Symptom Manag. 2017;54:231–6.
58. Nakagawa S, Ando M, Takayama H, et al. Withdrawal of left ventricular assist devices: a retrospective analysis from a single institution. J Palliat Med. 2020;23:368–74.
59. Brush S, Budge D, Alharethi R, et al. End-of-life decision making and implementation in recipients of a destination left ventricular assist device. J Heart Lung Transplant. 2010;29:1337–41.
60. Muhandiramge D, Udeoji DU, Biswas OS, et al. Palliative care issues in heart transplant candidates. Curr Opin Support Palliat Care. 2015;9:5–13.
61. Forsberg A, Lorenzon U, Nilsson F, Bäckmana L. Pain and health related quality of life after heart, kidney, and liver transplantation. Clin Transpl. 1999;13:453–60.

62. Holtzman S, Abbey SE, Stewart DE, Ross HJ. Pain after heart transplantation: prevalence and implications for quality of life. Psychosomatics. 2010;51:230–6.
63. Pudlo R, Piegza M, Zakliczyński M, Zembala M. The occurrence of mood and anxiety disorders in heart transplant recipients. Transplant Proc. 2009;41:3214–8.
64. Westerdahl AK, Sjöblom J, Mattiasson AC, Rosenqvist M, Frykman V. Implantable cardioverter-defibrillator therapy before death: high risk for painful shocks at end of life. Circulation. 2014;129:422–9.
65. Herman M, Horner K, Ly J, Vayl Y. Deactivation of implantable cardioverter-defibrillators in heart failure. J Hosp Palliat Nurs. 2018;20:63–71.
66. Sherazi S, McNitt S, Aktas MK, et al. End-of-life care in patients with implantable cardioverter defibrillators: a MADIT-II substudy. PACE Pacing Clin Electrophysiol. 2013;36:1273–9.
67. Costanzo MR, Mills RM, Wynne J. Characteristics of "Stage D" heart failure: insights from the Acute Decompensated Heart Failure National Registry Longitudinal Module (ADHERE LM). Am Heart J. 2008;155:339–47.
68. Chuzi S, Molsberry R, Ogunseitan A, et al. Trends in place of death for cardiovascular mortality related to heart failure in the United States from 2003 to 2017. Circ Heart Fail. 2020;13(2):e006587. https://doi.org/10.1161/CIRCHEARTFAILURE.119.006587.
69. Skorstengaard MH, Neergaard MA, Andreassen P, et al. Preferred place of care and death in terminally ill patients with lung and heart disease compared to cancer patients. J Palliat Med. 2017;20:1217–24.
70. Yancy CW, Jessup M, Bozkurt B, et al. 2017 ACC/AHA/HFSA focused update of the 2013 ACCF/AHA guideline for the management of heart failure: a report of the American College of Cardiology/American Heart Association task force on clinical practice guidelines and the Heart Failure Society of America. J Am Coll Cardiol. 2017;23:628–51.
71. Ponikowski P, Voors AA, Anker SD, et al. ESC guidelines for the diagnosis and treatment of acute and chronic heart failure. Eur Heart J. 2016;14(37):2129–200.
72. MacIver J, Wentlandt K, Ross HJ. Measuring quality of life in advanced heart failure. Curr Opin Support Palliat Care. 2017;11:12–6.
73. Packer M, Colucci W, Fisher L, et al. Effect of levosimendan on the short-term clinical course of patients with acutely decompensated heart failure. JACC Hear Fail. 2013;1:103–11.
74. Cuffe MS, Califf RM, Adams KF, et al. Short-term intravenous milrinone for acute exacerbation of chronic heart failure: a randomized controlled trial. J Am Med Assoc. 2002;287:1541–7.
75. Packer M, Carver JR, Rodeheffer RJ, et al. Effect of oral milrinone on mortality in severe chronic heart failure. The PROMISE Study Research Group. N Engl J Med. 1991;325:1468–75.
76. Nizamic T, Murad MH, Allen LA, et al. Ambulatory inotrope infusions in advanced heart failure: a systematic review and meta-analysis. JACC Heart Fail. 2018;6:757–67.
77. Crespo-Leiro MG, Metra M, Lund LH, et al. Advanced heart failure: a position statement of the Heart Failure Association of the European Society of Cardiology. Eur J Heart Fail. 2018;20:1505–35.
78. Hershberger RE, Nauman D, Walker TL, Dutton D, Burgess D. Care processes and clinical outcomes of continuous outpatient support with inotropes (COSI) in patients with refractory end-stage heart failure. J Card Fail. 2003;9:180–7.
79. Nanas JN, Tsagalou EP, Kanakakis J, et al. Long-term intermittent dobutamine infusion, combined with oral amiodarone for end-stage heart failure: a randomized double-blind study. Chest. 2004;125(4):1198–204. https://doi.org/10.1378/chest.125.4.1198.
80. Acharya D, Sanam K, Revilla-Martinez M, et al. Infections, arrhythmias, and hospitalizations on home intravenous inotropic therapy. Am J Cardiol. 2016;117(6):952–6. https://doi.org/10.1016/j.amjcard.2015.12.030.
81. Hashim T, Sanam K, Revilla-Martinez M, et al. Clinical characteristics and outcomes of intravenous inotropic therapy in advanced heart failure. Circ Hear Fail. 2015 Sep;8(5):880–6. https://doi.org/10.1161/CIRCHEARTFAILURE.114.001778.
82. Gorodeski EZ, Chu EC, Reese JR, Shishehbor MH, Hsich E, Starling RC. Prognosis on chronic dobutamine or milrinone infusions for stage D heart failure. Circ Heart Fail. 2009;2(4):320–4. https://doi.org/10.1161/CIRCHEARTFAILURE.108.839076.

83. Nieminen MS, Fonseca C, Brito D, Wikström G. The potential of the inodilator levosimendan in maintaining quality of life in advanced heart failure. Eur Heart J Suppl. 2017;19(Suppl C):C15–21.
84. Unverferth DV, Blanford M, Kates RE, Leier CV. Tolerance to dobutamine after a 72 hour continuous infusion. Am J Med. 1980;69(2):262–6. https://doi.org/10.1016/0002-9343(80)90387-3.
85. Malotte K, Saguros A, Groninger H. Continuous cardiac inotropes in patients with end-stage heart failure: an evolving experience. J Pain Symptom Manag. 2018;55(1):159–63. https://doi.org/10.1016/j.jpainsymman.2017.09.026.
86. Chuzi S, Allen LA, Dunlay SM, Warraich HJ. Palliative inotrope therapy: a narrative review. JAMA Cardiol. 2019;4(8):815–22. https://doi.org/10.1001/jamacardio.2019.2081.
87. Hauptman PJ, Mikolajczak P, George A, et al. Chronic inotropic therapy in end-stage heart failure. Am Heart J. 2006;152(6):1096.e1–8. https://doi.org/10.1016/j.ahj.2006.08.003.

Symptom Assessment and Management

3

Massimo Romanò

3.1 The Cardiologist's Palliative Competencies

Intensive care cardiologists operating in CICUs should have basic palliative care education and training [1]. That means being able to identify and provide basic treatment of symptoms (especially pain, dyspnea, anxiety, and depression), and discuss the treatment goals (in line with the patient's preferences), prognosis, advance directives (relating to end-of-life [EOL] choices), and eventual need for cardiopulmonary resuscitation.

Palliative care specialists, on the other hand, are certified professionals with competence in the palliative field. Specialists will be consulted in cooperation with the care team. Consultations deal with treatment of refractory pain and more complex forms of anxiety and depression; other debilitating symptoms such as dyspnea; suitable dosage and methods for opioid administration; discussion of existential issues; and assistance for the resolution of possible conflicts among family members or between family members and the care team.

Finally yet importantly is the discussion and management relating to palliative sedation at the EOL, a topic with a dedicated chapter in this book.

Symptoms can be pre-existing or new onset, both physical and psychological, especially in the final months/weeks before death [2].

Sometimes symptoms are caused by ongoing therapies (pharmacological or non-pharmacological) greatly impacting the patient's quality of life [3]. These are not the subject of the cardiologist's attention, which is focused on other specific problems, especially in the acute stages of the disease.

Patients requiring palliative care who are admitted or can potentially be admitted to CICU may suffer from different clinical problems. They can suffer from acute

M. Romanò (✉)
Organizing Committee, Postgraduate Master In Palliative Care, University of Milan, Milano, Italy
e-mail: max.romano51@gmail.com

M. Romanò (ed.), *Palliative Care in Cardiac Intensive Care Units*, https://doi.org/10.1007/978-3-030-80112-0_3

cardiovascular diseases [4] and they need palliative support during decision-making relating to possible treatment options.

Moreover, they could present severe symptoms and with fatal prognosis, they may evolve towards cardiogenic shock complicating an acute coronary syndrome, requiring mechanical circulatory support, as left ventricular assist device—LVAD [5].

Finally they may be affected by chronic cardiovascular disease.

This last case deals with patients who have previously shown acute stages of the disease and present a progressive deterioration of their general clinical conditions, associated with old age, multiple comorbidities, lung infection, or sepsis.

Patients suffering from advanced heart failure [6] are the most frequent. They present many concomitant symptoms at high intensity [3, 7–9].

The importance of identifying and treating symptoms, as well as those secondary to the underlying disease, has an important role since palliative care is an addition and not a replacement to treatment of the underlying disease and is not relevant only to terminally ill patients [10].

The most common symptoms are dyspnea, pain, depression, weakness, nausea, and sleeping disorders. The more these symptoms are present, the more life support, aggressive medical treatments, and intensive care admission are used.

Patients with cardiovascular diseases, especially with advanced heart failure, present a range of symptoms that are similar to cancer patients; however, these are less frequently assessed and treated. This means that patients with advanced heart failure have the same palliative needs as cancer patients [11].

3.2 Measuring a Symptom

A symptom is a subjective experience that is patient dependent. Therefore, it is difficult to identify one specific measuring scale related to the disease severity that is objective. Symptoms such as dyspnea or fatigue can be referred differently by patients according to the individual's ability to carry out a specific activity. This ability changes according to personal, environmental, social, and psychological conditions, and to the symptom perception, not merely to the disability induced by heart disease.

Whatever the symptom detection instrument used, it must be reliable (reproducible), valid (measuring the symptom), and sensitive (identifying symptom variations).

Unidimensional scales analyse one single variable: the specific symptom in question. This is a single parameter, where only intensity varies. Multidimensional scales analyse more elements at the same time; they are able to modulate the symptom's perception (sensorial, emotive, behavioural, motivational, sentimental, cognitive, social), but are more complex to use, compared to unidimensional scales. The choice of scale depends on the aim of the test, the clinical context (acute or chronic stage of a disease), and the examined population. Multidimensional scales detect various components of a symptom, whereas unidimensional scales belong to the

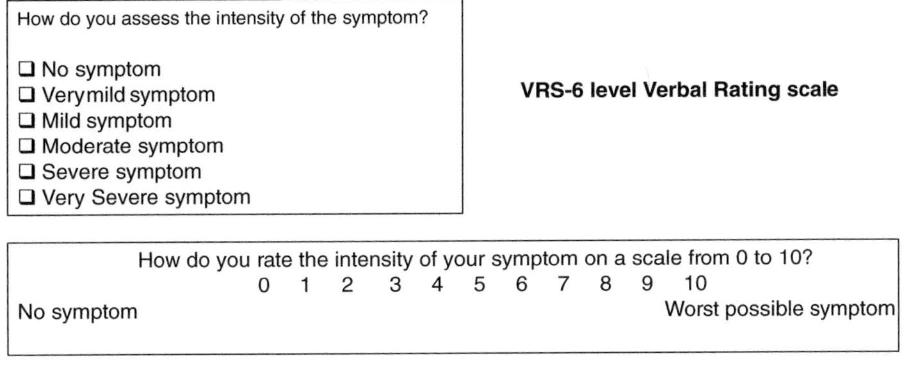

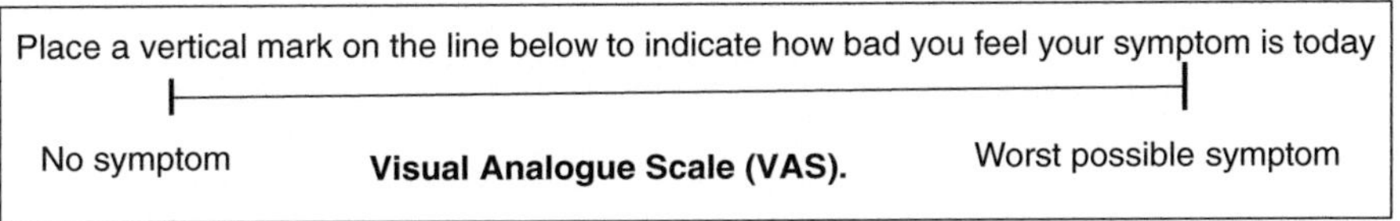

11 level Numerical Rating Scale (NRS).

Fig. 3.1 Unidimensional symptom rating scales

general set of clinical assessment tools of a patient, together with symptom variation assessment over time.

Unidimensional scales include verbal scales, numerical scales, and visual analogue scales, generally developed for pain assessment, and subsequently also used for other symptoms (see Fig. 3.1).

1. The Verbal Rating Scale (VRS) uses a set of verbal descriptors of the symptom ranging from "No symptom" to "Very severe symptom"; the descriptors are associated to numbers, corresponding to symptom intensity levels. There are generally six levels [12].
2. The Numerical Rating Scale (NRS) uses 11 levels, from 0, no symptom, to 11, the worst symptom possible [13].
3. The Visual Analogue Scale [VAS] uses a 10 cm horizontal or vertical line, on which only the two extreme values are indicated: "No symptom" and "Worst symptom possible". The patient is asked to mark the point that corresponds to the intensity of the symptom perceived at that moment. The score, ranging from 0 to 100, is measured in millimetres from the minimum intensity point to the point marked by the patient [14].

Symptom assessment can also employ the Likert scale that measures attitude and behaviour through a series of answer options that range from one extreme to another (e.g. from "improbable" to "extremely probable") [15].

Table 3.1 ESAS Scale—Edmonton Symptom Assessment System. From AHS Edmonton Zone Palliative Care Program, Covenant Health (CH) Palliative Institute & University of Alberta, with permission [16]

Pain	No pain	0	1	2	3	4	5	6	7	8	9	10	Worst possible pain
Tiredness	No tiredness	0	1	2	3	4	5	6	7	8	9	10	Worst possible tiredness
Nausea	No nausea	0	1	2	3	4	5	6	7	8	9	10	Worst possible nausea
Depression	No depression	0	1	2	3	4	5	6	7	8	9	10	Worst possible depression
Anxiety	No anxiety	0	1	2	3	4	5	6	7	8	9	10	Worst possible anxiety
Drowsiness	No drowsiness	0	1	2	3	4	5	6	7	8	9	10	Worst possible drowsiness
Anorexia	No anorexia	0	1	2	3	4	5	6	7	8	9	10	Worst possible anorexia
Well-being	Best well-being	0	1	2	3	4	5	6	7	8	9	10	Worst possible well-being
Dyspnea	No dyspnea	0	1	2	3	4	5	6	7	8	9	10	Worst possible dyspnea
Other	No symptom	0	1	2	3	4	5	6	7	8	9	10	Worst possible symptom

The Edmonton Symptom Assessment Scale (ESAS and its revised version ESASr) is a relatively simple scale to use, developed for everyday assessment of cancer patients' symptoms, while undergoing palliative care [16]. Its original version is also applicable to non-cancer patients, such as heart failure patients admitted to ICU and with high risk of death [17]. It allows an overall assessment of patient quality of life. It is made up of nine visual numeric scales (from 0 to 10) for the following symptoms: pain, fatigue, nausea, depression, anxiety, drowsiness, anorexia, general malaise, and dyspnea. There is also a tenth, optional symptom that can be added by the patient, shown as "other" (Table 3.1). There is a good correlation between ESAS, the New York Heart Association (NYHA) functional classification, and the Kansas City Cardiomyopathy Questionnaire (KCCQ).

Behavioural scales are used when the patient is unconscious or unable to communicate symptoms autonomously. These allow assessment and measurement of reaction to symptoms (especially dyspnea and pain).

3.2.1 Dyspnea

A consensus statement from the American Thoracic Society offers a definition: "Dyspnea is a term used to characterise a subjective experience of breathing discomfort that is composed of qualitatively distinct sensations that vary in intensity. The experience derives from interactions among multiple physiological, psychological, social, and environmental factors, and may induce secondary physiological and behavioral responses" [18].

Dyspnea is the main symptom of heart failure and chronic obstructive pulmonary disease (COPD) and is a common reason for access to health facilities.

Dyspnea has a variable prevalence but tends to be above 50%, especially in the last year of life, in different diseases [2], particularly in heart failure where it can peak at over 80% towards the last weeks [19], and generally in organ failure [20].

It is also among the prevalent symptoms in patients admitted to ICU, both for cancer (34%) [21] and advanced chronic diseases undergoing mechanical ventilation (47–60%) [22, 23], or in patients with a high risk of death (44%) [17].

Dyspnea worsens functional capacity and quality of life, independently of disease severity.

Skeletal myopathy, which develops with heart failure as a consequence of chronic hemodynamic stress, also affects the respiratory muscles and diaphragm. It is considered a joint cause of dyspnea [24], together with anemia, COPD [25] often concurrent with heart failure, and obesity.

Of note is the correlation with inflammation markers, and above all, the correlation with psychological stress (depression and anxiety), aging, and disease severity.

In restrictive and obstructive (COPD) lung diseases the mechanisms are different and more complex [26].

The most common scales used for measuring dyspnea are the Numerical Rating Scale [27], the 4-level Verbal Descriptor Scale (none, mild, moderate, severe) which is similar to the Visual Analogue Scale [28], the modified Borg scale [29] (Table 3.2), the Medical Research Council scale (MRC) (Table 3.3) [30], and the Likert scale (Table 3.4) [31].

Around one-third of critically ill patients admitted to ICU are unable to communicate their symptoms, using the abovementioned scales [32]. For this reason, the 8-parameter ordinal Respiratory Distress Observation Scale (RODS) is used [32], also validated in ICU [17] (Table 3.5). From 0 to 2 points there is no distress, 3 points means mild distress, from 4 to 6 moderate, and >7 severe distress [32].

Table 3.2 Modified 0–10 Borg scale. From Kendrick with permission [29]

Borg scale (modified) for dyspnea	
0.	No breathlessness at all
0.5	Very, very slight (just noticeable)
1.	Very slight
2.	Slight breathlessness
3.	Moderate
4.	Somewhat severe
5.	Severe breathlessness
6.	
7.	Very severe breathlessness
8.	
9.	Very, very severe (almost maximal)
10.	Maximal

Table 3.3 MRC dyspnea assessment scale. Used with the permission of the Medical Research Council [30]

MRC scale for dyspnea
Grade 1: I only get breathless with strenuous exercise
Grade 2: I get short of breath when hurrying on the level or up a slight hill
Grade 3: I walk slower than people of the same age on the level because of breathlessness or have to stop for breath when walking at my own pace on the level
Grade 4: I stop for breath after walking 100 yards or after a few minutes on the level
Grade 5: I am too breathless to leave the house

Table 3.4 Likert scale to measure dyspnea. Modified with permission from Pang [31]

5	The worst breathlessness possible
4	Severe breathlessness
3	Moderate breathlessness
2	Mild breathlessness
1	No breathlessness at all

Table 3.5 Respiratory Distress Observation Scale—RDOS. From Campbell [32], with permission

Variables	0 point	1 point	2 points	Total
Heart rate per minute	<90 beats	90–109 beats	>110 beats	
Respiratory rate per minute	≤18 breaths	19-30 breaths	>30 breaths	
Restlessness: nonpurposeful movements	None	Occasional, slight movements	Frequent movements	
Accessory muscle use: rise in clavicle in inspiration	None	Slight rise	Pronounced rise	
Paradoxical breathing pattern: abdomen moves in on inspiration	None		Present	
Grunting at end-expiration: guttural sound	None		Present	
Nasal flaring: involuntary movement of nares	None		Present	
Look of fear	None		Eyes wide open, facial muscles tense, brow furrowed, mouth open	
Total				

The main goal of therapy is based on the optimization of pharmacological and non-pharmacological treatment of the underlying diseases, especially advanced heart failure [6].

Despite this, dyspnea can persist and affect the quality of life, above all in the most advanced stages of heart failure and near death; therefore it must be suitably treated.

Various treatment procedures have been suggested to reduce dyspnea:

1. Maintaining patient posture to minimize dyspnea perception [32].
2. Non-pharmacological procedures such as the use of a handheld fan [33].
3. Additional oxygen support: This is often used in various ways and has a palliative aim in patients in the advanced stages of disease. Oxygen support is delivered either with the traditional method or with a high-flow nasal cannula, or with noninvasive ventilation.

   Clinical results show that in case of stable COPD and hypoxemia the application of these procedures is linked to a reduction in mortality.

   On the other hand, clinical results related to patients in the advanced stages of heart or lung disease with dyspnea but no hypoxemia are controversial.

   The medical procedure that seems to be more effective in the control of dyspnea is ventilation with high-flow nasal cannula [33].
4. Opioids, administered orally or intravenously, are the first-choice treatment for patients presenting dyspnea and advanced diseases: available data refers mainly to patients with COPD and cancer and shows efficacy in alleviating the symptom, without significant increase in important side effects, such as respiratory depression, nor any acceleration of death in EOL patients. Data is more contradictory when it comes to the use of opioids in patients with advanced heart failure and refractory dyspnea, due to the inferior number of cases examined [32, 33].

   Despite there not being clear scientific evidence [34] the guidelines recommend their use [33].

   Opioids act via different mechanisms: reduction in the respiratory drive, change in dyspnea central perception, decrease in peripheral pulmonary receptor activity, and anxiety reduction [32].

   When dosing starts low and is titrated slowly upwards, there is good evidence for a reduction in dyspnea. Morphine is the most commonly used opioid.

   In patients already being treated with opioids for pain (tolerant patients) dosages are gradually increased up to 25–50% of the current daily dose.

   Morphine should be used for acute, intense dyspnea, and in the terminal stages of disease. It should be administered via intravenous bolus, and then via continuous infusion, modulating doses according to symptom control, or subcutaneously with equivalent dosages, checking the achieved level of sedation with the Richmond Agitation-Sedation Scale (RASS) [35, 36] (Table 3.6).

   The initial intravenous/subcutaneous dose, in naive patients, can be 2–2.5 mg, with an effect assessment within about 15 min; if dyspnea persists, another dose can be administered and, when the symptoms have been brought under control, maintain a 5 mg administration every 4 h or with continuous infusion at 2 mg/h. If side effects such as nausea or marked constipation appear, move to 0.5 mg intravenous/subcutaneous hydromorphone administration every 4 h [37].

   Table 3.7 lists the molecules and recommended dosages for the control of dyspnea in naive patients.

Table 3.6 RASS scale. From Laerkner et al., with permission [35]

Richmond agitation-sedation scale

	Target RASS value	RASS description
+4	Combative	Combative, violent, immediate danger to staff
+3	Very Agitated	Pulls or removes tube(s) or catheter(s); aggressive
+2	Agitated	Frequent non-purposeful movement, fights ventilator
+1	Restless	Anxious, apprehensive but movements are not aggressive or vigorous
0	Alert and Calm	
−1	Drowsy	Not fully alert, but has sustained awakening to voice (eye opening & contact **greater** than 10 s)
−2	Light Sedation	Briefly awakens to voice (eye opening & contact **less** than 10 s)
−3	Moderate Sedation	Movements or eye opening to voice (but **NO** eye contact)
−4	Deep Sedation	No response to voice, *but* has movement or eye opening to physical stimulation
−5	Unarousable	No response to voice or physical stimulation

Table 3.7 Opioid dosage in the treatment of refractory dyspnea in opioid-naive patients. *IV* Intravenous, *SC* Subcutaneous. Adapted from Pisani [33], with permission

Opioid	IV/SC dose—adult
Morphine sulfate	2–2.5 mg in bolus/3–4 h—IV/SC 5 mg/4 h maintenance dose 2 mg/h IV continuous infusion
Hydromorphone	0.5 mg–1 mg/3–4 h—IV/SC
Fentanyl	25–50 µg/h IV

When the patient has been clinically stabilized, oral administration instead of the intravenous/subcutaneous route can eventually be considered, respecting the 1:3 conversion rate in determining daily dosage.

Dosages are modified according to liver and kidney functioning.

5. If anxiety and panic occur due to dyspnea, benzodiazepines can be administered, although evidence to support their action in reducing dyspnea is not solid and recommendations are based on observational studies [33].

    Benzodiazepines must be considered after opioids or other medication. Oral and sublingual lorazepam (0.5–1 mg) and intravenous or subcutaneous midazolam (1–2.5 mg), that in severe dyspnea can be given via continuous infusion (10–20 mg/day) with or without associated morphine [32], are the drugs used until the desired effect is achieved.

    There is no evidence that non-opioid-based pharmacological therapies (selective serotonin reuptake inhibitors, tricyclic antidepressants) are effective.

6. There is no data supporting the palliative use of corticosteroids, when severe COPD is excluded [33].

Slawnych [37] states five aspects to remember in EOL patients with dyspnea:

1. No one must die suffering from dyspnea.
2. Opioids are first-choice treatment.
3. If symptoms persist, also give benzodiazepines.
4. In the final stage, bothersome secretions interfering with deglutition may appear. Use subcutaneous scopolamine, 0.4 mg every 4 h, increasing the dosage until the symptom is under control, or subcutaneous hyoscine butylbromide starting from 20 mg to a maximum dosage of 100 mg in 24 h. Pay attention to the sedative effect. Alternatively, if the drugs are ineffective or sedation is excessive, subcutaneous or intravenous glycopyrrolate can be given 0.2/0.4 mg every 4 h. Remember the anticholinergic side effect.
5. Treat family members' agitation due to the patient's dyspnea.

3.2.2   Pain

Pain is defined as "an unpleasant sensory and emotional experience associated with actual or potential tissue damage, or described in terms of such damage" [38].

Pain is a frequent symptom in patients with chronic diseases and in patients with advanced heart failure where it is often underestimated and undertreated.

Pain was the most relevant symptom assessed in a clinical study conducted on 4700 patients who died from different diseases, and who were evaluated during the last 2 years of life. The study reports that 46% of patients with heart disease suffered from moderate-severe intensity pain [39].

In the PAIN-HF study, 80% of patients with advanced heart failure experienced pain; in one-third of cases this was located in multiple sites [40].

The origin can be somatic (musculoskeletal), visceral, or neuropathic, located mainly in the inferior limbs, spinal column, and shoulders. The incidence of cardiac pain does not exceed 20–30% of cases [40].

Pain was registered in 57–75% in another series of patients with advanced heart failure within the last 6 months of life [2, 19].

Pain intensity correlates to psychological, social, and spiritual aspects, highlighting the often multifactorial nature of pain [41].

There is no attributable data for CICU patients.

So, references are only possible to ICU patients [17], where 40% register moderate-severe pain intensity, not infrequently during procedures (Table 3.8) [38].

The standard pain assessment scales, when self-reported, are VRS [12], NRS [13], and VAS [14] (see Fig. 3.1).

Behavioral scales can be used both in the assessment stages and after specific treatment, when dealing with patients that are unable to communicate (because of intubation, sedation, or delirium).

The most common and validated behavioral scales in ICU (in patients where behavior is observable) are the Behavioral Pain Scale in intubated (BPS) and non-intubated (BPS-NI) patients (which analyze facial expression, upper limb movements, and compliance to mechanical ventilation) and the Critical Care Pain Observation Tool (CPOT), which analyzes facial expression, body movement,

Table 3.8 Painful procedures in ICU

Arterial line insertion
Central intravenous line insertion
Peripheral intravenous line insertion
Peripheral venous and arterial blood draws
Femoral sheet removal
Pericardial or pleural drain insertion
Urine catheter insertion
Respiratory exercises
Mobilization, turning, and repositioning
Nasogastric tube insertion
Tracheal suctioning
Extubation
Nursing care procedures

muscle tension, compliance to ventilator in intubated patients, and vocalization in non-intubated patients. Another scale is Behavior Pain Assessment Tool (BPAT) [38, 42].

Assessment scales based on physiological variables, such as cardiac or breathing frequency, are not sufficiently validated.

In CICU patients with noncardiac pain, pharmacological treatment must be based on the correct diagnosis of the type of pain, nociceptive, neuropathic, or mixed, as these are treated with different drugs.

To this aim, the combined skills of the cardiologist and palliative care specialist are fundamental in obtaining the best possible results in terms of symptom intensity reduction.

The basic principle of pain treatment, as with other symptoms, is to employ effective medication at regular intervals, with a dosage that is suitable for the pain intensity, with particular attention to side effects.

For ICU patients experiencing pain, opioids are considered the first-line drugs. However, due to their side effects (sedation, delirium, respiratory depression, nausea, constipation, thirst) they can be used together with other pharmacological and non-pharmacological treatments to lower opioid dosage and to implement multimodal analgesia.

Non-opioid adjuvants suggested by the guidelines [39, 42] do not have a high level of evidence and are illustrated in Table 3.9.

Nonsteroidal anti-inflammatory drugs (NSAIDs) are forbidden in patients with heart failure due to their hydro-saline retention properties and heart failure deterioration.

Nociceptive pain will be treated with opioids, if paracetamol test proves ineffective [38].

Patients experiencing neuropathic pain can benefit from treatment with gabapentinoids or tricyclic antidepressants, with or without opioids [38, 43].

When pain is intense and refractory to adjuvants, intravenous/subcutaneous administration of opioids is advised, as in Table 3.10.

Table 3.9 Adjuvant drugs in pain relief. CKD: chronic kidney disease

Drug	Initial dose	Titration	Side effects
Paracetamol Nociceptive pain	1 g every 6 h IV	Adjust if hepatopathy or renal insufficiency	Arterial hypotension
Nefopam Periprocedural pain	20 mg IV/30 min		Tachycardia, vertigo, delirium
Gabapentin Neuropathic pain	300 mg od	300 mg bid 300 mg td Dose max 2.4 g/die	Vertigo, drowsiness, difficulty walking
Pregabalin Neuropathic pain	75 mg bid	Double every 3 days. Max dose 300 mg bid	Vertigo, drowsiness
Carbamazepine Neuropathic pain	200 mg od	Increase every 3 days up to 600 mg bid	Sedation, nausea, ataxia
Amitriptyline Neuropathic pain	10-25 mg at the bedtime	Increase every 3 days. Max dose 150 mg	Sedation, xerostomia
Duloxetine Neuropathic pain	15 mg od	Max dose 60 mg od Not advised in severe CKD	Arterial hypotension Tachycardia

Table 3.10 Opioid doses for pain control. *ER* Extended release, *TD* Transdermal, *IV* Intravenous, *SC* Subcutaneous, *po* oral

Drug	Starting IV/ SC dose	Maintenance IV/ SC dose	Half-life	Chronic dose
Morphine	2–5 mg bolus IV/SC	1–10 mg/h infusion	2–4 h	10-30mg/6h po or ER dose equivalent or maintain infusion
Hydromorphone	1-2 mg IV/ SC /3-4 h	IV 0.1-0.4 mg h infusion	2-3 h	0.5-1 mg/3-4h po or ER 8-32 mg/24 h or maintain infusion
Fentanyl	25–100 µg bolus	25–200 µg/h infusion	2–5 h	25-100 µg/h/72h TD or mantain infusion
Ramifentanyl	0.5–2 mg bolus	0.5–15 µg/kg/h infusion	3–10 min	NA

In opioid-naive patients start with the lower range dose, increasing progressively to reach the best analgesic result. Then start with maintenance dose.

As previously mentioned dosages are gradually increased to 25–50% for the simultaneous treatment of pain in patients that are already being treated with opioids (tolerant patients).

When oral route of administration is possible, in naive patients it is best to start with low doses of short-acting drugs until the effective daily dose required for pain control is assessed. The transition from short-acting to long-acting will be then further assessed, tailoring therapy strategy to meet the desired effect and the patient's needs, at equivalent doses.

There are many opioid molecules and formulations available for oral treatment. These are grouped according to their duration of action:

1. Long-acting opioids (LAO): Long-acting morphine sulfate, long-acting oxycodone, hydromorphone, methadone, transdermal fentanyl, and transdermal buprenorphine. These have a latency to peak effect of 1–3 h and duration of action of about 12 h or more (i.e., transdermal fentanyl or buprenorphine).
2. Short-acting opioids (SAO): Morphine solution (immediate-release morphine), oxycodone, buprenorphine, tramadol, codeine. These have a latency to peak effect of 30–40 min and duration of action of about 4 h.
3. Rapid-onset opioids (ROO): Fentanyl in various rapid transmucosal absorption formulations (i.e., nasal, buccal, sublingual). Latency to peak effect of 15 min and duration of action of around 2 h. Indicated in breakthrough cancer pain—BTcP.

When passing from morphine to other opioids or vice versa, dosage is determined using conversion tables.

The opioids' main side effects are shown in Table 3.11.

Transmucosal or transdermal route of administration can be used in patients that are unable to swallow.

A special attention should be addressed to treat periprocedural pain in CICU: opioids, impromptu NSAIDs, and volatile anesthetics are suggested [38].

3.2.3 Thirst

Thirst has been defined as "the sensation that leads animal and human actions toward the goal of finding and drinking water [44]."

Thirst, which often accompanies xerostomia, is a frequent and underestimated symptom, with a 70% prevalence in patients admitted to ICU [45].

It is described by patients as an important symptom, above all during fluid restriction during recurrences of heart failure, and is disabling, ultimately affecting the quality of life [17].

It is experienced in 20% of patients with chronic heart failure; this figure triples in the recurrent stages [46] and tends to persist in around 15% of patients [47].

Thirst in ICU patients is mainly linked to underlying disease severity, expressed by a higher APACHE II score, and above all to high dosages of opioids ($\geq$50 mg/

Table 3.11 Main opioid side effects

Drug	Main side effects
Morphine	Hypotension, bradycardia, nausea, vomiting, constipation, drowsiness
Hydromorphone	Nausea, vomiting, dizziness, headache, drowsiness
Fentanyl	Nausea, vomiting, constipation, drowsiness
Ramifentanyl	Bradycardia, hypotension

Table 3.12 Thirst Distress Scale (TDS-HF) for patients with heart failure. From Waldreus et al [49], with permission

Statement	Strongly disagree				Strongly agree
1. My thirst bothers me a lot	1	2	3	4	5
2. I am very uncomfortable when I am thirsty	1	2	3	4	5
3. My mouth feels like sandpaper when I am thirsty	1	2	3	4	5
4. My mouth feels dry when I am thirsty	1	2	3	4	5
5. My saliva is very thin when I am thirsty	1	2	3	4	5
6. When I drink less water, my thirst gets worse	1	2	3	4	5
7. I am so thirsty I could drink water uncontrollably	1	2	3	4	5
8. My thirst feels difficult to overcome	1	2	3	4	5

day), and furosemide (>60 mg/day), serotonin reuptake inhibitor use, and low levels of ionized calcium [48].

An explanation for this last point could be the presence of calcium-sensitive brain receptors, involved in the central regulation of fluids and electrolyte balance [48].

Other factors that might induce thirst are administration of benzodiazepines, tolvaptan used for the treatment of hyponatremia, and activation of the renin–angiotensin–aldosterone system [47].

Fluid restriction and associated gastrointestinal pathologies are predictors of symptom intensity, whereas secondary thirst distress is associated with mechanical ventilation, negative fluid balance, and antihypertensive medication [48].

Thirst can be measured via VAS, NRS, and TDS (Thirst Distress Scale) [49] (Table 3.12).

TDS is a 5-point Likert scale, with 8 items relating to thirst in heart failure patients. The patient is questioned on the characteristics of their thirst and expresses greater or lesser agreement on every item, from 1 (completely disagree) to 5 (completely agree). The total score can vary from 8 to 40. The higher the score, the greater the symptom intensity. Scores from 8 to 16 express absence of the symptom or light symptom, and 17 to 40 express moderate-severe symptom [49].

Other than eventual treatment variation, there is no specific treatment for thirst except for cold sterile water sprays, cold sterile water swabs, use of mouth and lip moisturizer, and peppermint-flavor chewing gum [50, 51].

3.3 Cognitive and Mood Disorders

Pain, agitation, and delirium are the "ICU triad" [38].

Agitation, defined as the state of excessive psychomotor activity accompanied by tension and irritability, affects 55–59% of ICU patients [52].

It may often require sedative treatment to reduce stress (this applies mainly to patients undergoing mechanical ventilation) and to reduce complication from any potential patient self-harm [38].

Medication for agitation must be aimed at the lightest sedation possible (even if there is no consensus on the definition of "light sedation"), avoiding the use of benzodiazepines and opioids as much as possible, as they could provoke delirium and prolong mechanical ventilation and ICU length of stay (LOS) [38].

Propofol and dexmedetomidine are drugs with equivalent efficacy that should be privileged during mechanical ventilation and delirium, even if dexmedetomidine registered a lower incidence of delirium in one trial [38].

Dexmedetomidine is an $alpha_2$ presynaptic adrenergic agonist, with sedative, sympatholytic, amnesiac, and analgesic effects: it is short-acting.

The dosage used in a far-reaching study of 2000 patients was 1 µg/kg/h without initial bolus, with a maximum dose of 1.4 µg/kg/h; it can also be used after an initial bolus of 0.7 µg/kg/h, with a maintenance dosage varying from 0.2 to 1.4 µg/kg/h and adjusted to the planned level of sedation [53].

In a recent multicenter Spanish trial [54] carried out on over 400 patients admitted to third-level CICU, of which 53% underwent mechanical ventilation, the drug showed a low percentage of early reintubation (1.7%), suggesting a benefit in ventilation weaning. However, other sedatives had to be administered to 85% of patients, showing that this medication alone does not allow deep sedation.

Essentially dexmedetomidine can be proposed for moderate sedation (RASS from 0 to −3), allowing better patient management and communication, whereas propofol/midazolam are advised for deep and prolonged sedation [55]. Dexmedetomidine might be used in procedural sedation, not uncommon in CICU, with dosages of 1 µg/kg in 10 min, followed by a maintenance infusion of 0.6 µg/kg/h, adjusted to reach the desired effect with a dosage variable from 0.2 to 1 µg/kg/h.

These dosages decrease when dealing with old or frail patients.

With deep or prolonged sedation, the suggested dosages for midazolam and propofol vary, ranging from 0.03 to 0.2 mg/kg/h for midazolam and from 0.3 to 4.0 mg/kg/h for propofol [55].

****

Preexisting cognitive deficit, especially dementia, is present in about 40% of ICU patients. The main factors that predict preexisting cognitive deficit are age (>65 years), sex (higher incidence in females), being single, and disease severity measured with the APACHE II score [56]. Prevalence of cognitive deficit varies between 25% and 50% in heart failure patients, according to the diagnostic test used. It is characterized by diminished levels of attention, reduced thought processing speed, and memory loss. Reduced cardiac output and cerebrovascular disease can be the main causes [57].

Heart failure patients risk developing significant cognitive deficit more than individuals without heart failure; cognitive deficit relates to higher mortality and a higher risk of developing dementia [58].

Delirium is closely linked to cognitive disorders: delirium and dementia are frequent causes of cognitive deterioration, especially in elderly patients. These can be independent, but often coexist [59].

Dementia is the main risk factor in delirium development.

"Delirium is a state of an acute disturbance of awareness and attention that commonly arises during critical disease; the syndrome represents a decompensation of cerebral function in response to one or more pathophysiological stressors" [59].

Its acute onset is accompanied with disorders of memory, attention, language, thought processing, and behavioral, together with possible hallucinatory phases.

The prevalence of delirium depends on the examined population: it varies from 0.4 to 2% in the community, and it is around 20% in hospitalized patients, especially in the elderly and during acute stages of disease, affecting around 80% of patients assisted by mechanical ventilation or at the end of life [60].

Delirium frequency varies from 8.3 to 28.8% in CICU patients, in relation to the type of diagnostic tests used [61–64].

Interestingly a study conducted in two Italian CICUs, on around 500 patients older than 65 years (average age 79 years), reported delirium in 18% of cases, half of which appeared within 24 h of admission (prevalent delirium).

Indicators of delirium development are advanced age, acute respiratory distress, ST-segment elevation myocardial infarction, comorbidities, disease severity, and dementia [61].

Delirium impacts in-hospital mortality from 17% to 33% [65], significantly higher than patients without delirium (27% vs. 3%) [59], and longer lengths of stay [65].

Regarding the link between delirium and adverse outcomes, it is still not clear whether it is a cause or simply a marker of elevated risk [66].

Two studies reported mortality at 6 months from CICU discharge: a prospective one, dealing with patients consecutively admitted to CICU for different reasons (54.9% vs. 8.9% of patients without delirium) [61], and a retrospective one dealing with 1,333,000 patients following acute myocardial infarction (10.5% vs. 7.6%) [67].

Delirium is a multifactorial syndrome, with many underlying causes. It results from the interaction of predisposing conditions (advanced age, cognitive deficit, disease severity, dementia) and precipitating conditions. The most important delirium precipitating conditions in ICUs, and especially in CICUs, are:

1. Drug administration, mainly opioids, benzodiazepines, antidepressants, anticholinergics, antivirals, some antiarrhythmic like procainamide and amiodarone, and digoxin [65].
2. Advanced age (>65): 9–44% of aging individuals with cardiovascular disease risk developing delirium in ICU, particularly if already affected by cognitive disorders or preexisting sensory disturbances [68].
3. Organ failure, especially heart failure (up to 30% of cases), infection, malnutrition, dehydration, pain, anxiety, presence of intravenous/intra-arterial/bladder catheters, frequent blood samples [61].
4. Pain of any cause.
5. Invasive procedures: mechanical ventilation, temporary cardiac pacing, mechanical circulatory support, transcatheter aortic valve implantation—TAVI [64, 65].
6. Cardiogenic shock and acute renal failure [62].

7. High disease severity, measured with APACHE II and SAPS II scores [62].
8. CICU environmental factors: noise (often coming from continuous alarms of monitoring systems—alarm fatigue), lights, presence or absence of windows, spatial isolation (box), family members visiting only at set times, bedbound, connection to monitor, oxygen mask, frequent assessment of vital signs are all factors that contribute to sleep deprivation. Fragmented sleep, caused by continuous impacting disturbances, is a determining factor for delirium development, longer duration of mechanical ventilation, altered immune system functioning, and neurocognitive dysfunction [38].

Although neglected, sleep disturbances are very frequent (up to 50% of cases) in patients admitted to ICU [68] and are often associated with mechanical and noninvasive ventilation [38].

Delirium can occur with three prevalent clinical pictures: the hyperactive type (characterized by hallucinations and psychomotor agitation), the hypoactive type (apathy, lethargy, sedation), and the mixed type.

According to literature the prevalence of the three types in ICU varies: the hypoactive type is classically considered the most frequent (65%), the hyperactive accounts for 25% of cases, and the mixed accounts for 10% [69].

However, on the basis of clinical records collected in Italian CICUs, the overall most common type appears to be the hyperactive one (63.1%), followed by the mixed (19.8%) and then the hypoactive one (12.6%) [61].

In a more recent systematic review and meta-analysis on delirium in ICU, the prevalence of the hypoactive type is 55%, the mixed type 32%, and the hyperactive 13% [70].

Two other clinical types have been described, a "catatonic" type which is an extreme form of the hypoactive type and an "excited" type which is an extreme form of the hyperactive type. The latter is often linked to sympathomimetic drug abuse, such as amphetamines [70].

Hypoactive delirium has a higher in-hospital CICU mortality rate (42.9%) compared to the hyperactive type (12.5%) and the mixed one (4.5%) [61].

The onset of delirium in ICU increases cognitive deterioration tenfold at discharge [71].

It is estimated that around 30–40% of delirium cases can be prevented with close assessment of possible causes [61]. However, even if greater attention is given to the early identification of delirium and to the correction of risk factors, there is little significant variation in the prevalence of delirium in ICU [38], which remains high.

From the diagnostic point of view, it is important to differentiate delirium from depression, psychosis, and dementia, which can all coexist [72].

Dementia is the main risk factor for delirium, which is diagnosed with the DSM-5 criteria [73]. The delirium assessment scale is expressed via various screening tests, the most common being CAM (Confusion Assessment Method) [74] (Table 3.13), adapted to ICU patients, and CAM-ICU [75], especially if undergoing mechanical ventilation, a procedure highly correlated to delirium (80% of patients) and impacting 30% of in-hospital mortality [60].

When dealing with unconscious or comatose patients, the Richmond Agitation-Sedation Scale 3 can be used, together with CAM [61]. Delirium is considered

Table 3.13 Confusion Assessment Method—CAM for delirium diagnosis. Modified from Inouye with permission [74]

The diagnosis of delirium requires the presence of both 1 and 2 and either 3 or 4
Feature 1. Acute onset and fluctuating course This feature is usually obtained from a family member or nurse and is shown by positive responses to the following questions: (a) Is there evidence of an acute change in mental status from the patient's baseline? (b) Did the (abnormal) behavior fluctuate during the day, that is, tend to come and go, or increase and decrease in severity?
Feature 2. Inattention This feature is shown by a positive response to the following question: Did the patient have difficulty focusing attention, for example, being easily distractible, or having difficulty keeping track of what was being said?
Feature 3. Disorganized thinking This feature is shown by a positive response to the following question: Was the patient's thinking disorganized or incoherent, such as rambling or irrelevant conversation, unclear or illogical flow of ideas, or unpredictable switching from subject to subject?
Feature 4. Altered level of consciousness (rated with RASS score) This feature is shown by any answer other than "alert" to the following question: Overall, how would you rate this patient's level of consciousness? (alert [normal], vigilant [hyperalert], lethargic [drowsy, easily aroused], stupor [difficult to arouse], or coma [unarousable])

prevalent if CAM assessment is positive within 24 h of admission, or incident if it appears after 24 h from admission [61].

Treatment of delirium must identify and address any trigger/predisposition causes previously listed. Treatment is pharmacological and non-pharmacological.

Non-pharmacological treatment of delirium is similar to the preventive one. It must be followed throughout hospitalization and is multifaceted [76]. It includes:

(a) Early mobilization, especially in elderly patients [38, 68].
(b) Space-time reorientation (for example, placing a clock in front of the patient's bed or using a calendar).
(c) Nursing station noise reduction.
(d) Lights on/off during the day/night cycle.
(e) The presence of windows.
(f) More frequent family access.
(g) Use of glasses and hearing equipment.
(h) Limitation of restraining devices.
(i) Nutrition and hydration improvement, treatment of infections.
(j) Treatment of sleep disorders (haloperidol, atypical antipsychotics such as risperidone, olanzapine, and quetiapine increase total sleep time and its quality [68], while melatonin has shown inconclusive results): Benzodiazepines are unadvised especially for the elderly due to the risk of developing adverse events, such as delirium or excessive sedation.

These measures allow adequate re-establishment of the sleep-wake cycle [38, 61].
However recent meta-analyses have cast doubt on the efficacy of the various non-pharmacological treatments in reducing the incidence and duration of delirium [76, 77].

Pharmacological therapy of delirium is mainly symptomatic and should be given when there is a risk to patient safety or when patients with hyperactive delirium cannot be treated with the proper therapies [76].

Firstly, the presence and intensity of pain and its suitable treatment need to be assessed.

Randomized clinical studies report a lack of clarity regarding the pharmacological efficacy of the drugs used to treat or prevent delirium, while some meta-analyses have offered controversial indications [78, 79].

Guidelines do not suggest the use of drugs for the prevention of delirium, as there is no sufficient clinical evidence, albeit low doses of dexmedetomidine at night have been indicated as able to reduce the incidence of delirium in ICU [38]. Melatonin (at an average dose of 3.5 mg) and its agonist ramelteon have recently been suggested for the prevention of delirium, with preliminary but promising results [78, 80].

Antipsychotics, particularly haloperidol, are still considered the first-choice treatment in the acute phase of delirium [78], even if not routinely given; according to the Society of Critical Care Medicine guidelines there is no clear evidence in the reduction of mechanical ventilation or ICU LOS [38].

When dealing with antipsychotics, it is important to consider the risk of developing adverse events associated to their use: extrapyramidal symptoms, sedation, anticholinergic effects, QT interval prolongation, and possible secondary ventricular arrhythmia, as well as interaction with other drugs.

Dexmedetomidine has shown to significantly reduce the duration of delirium, mechanical ventilation, and ICU hospitalization. To this purpose it has been suggested by the Society of Critical Care Medicine guidelines [38, 79] and has also been recently proposed in CICU with positive results [54, 65].

Among the atypical antipsychotic drugs, olanzapine, quetiapine, ziprasidone, and risperidone have been studied, also with contrasting results [65, 81–83].

The suggested dosages are reported in Table 3.14.

The use of benzodiazepine must be avoided, except in delirium due to alcohol withdrawal.

Nevertheless, a recent meta-analysis suggests the combined administration of 2 mg intravenous haloperidol and 3 mg intravenous lorazepam as the best treatment for agitation in the hyper-acute stages of delirium, rather than just haloperidol [78]. The use of haloperidol must be closely assessed in patients with acute myocardial infarction, as it induces a modest but significant increase in mortality when compared to other atypical antipsychotics, particularly in the first week of treatment [84].

Mood disorders in ICU (anxiety, sadness, depression, fear) are common, 35–58%, and negatively impact the quality of life in critically ill patients [45, 85].

In more detail, anxiety and depression range from 12% to 43% [86], and 10 to 30%, respectively, in patients admitted to ICU [87].

Another important psychological problem is post-traumatic stress disorder (PTSD), which can involve patients and family members, with high prevalence (20%) [88].

In these cases, effective communication with the patient/family members, aimed at limiting psychological disorders, is fundamental.

Table 3.14 Suggested drugs to treat delirium

Medication	Recommended dosage	Side effects	Contraindication	Evidence	Ref
Haloperidol	Oral: 0.5–5 mg every 6–8 h IV/IM 0.5–10 mg q15 to 30 min until response achieved, then give 25% of last bolus dose Q6H	QTc prolongation, extrapyramidal effects	Prolonged QTc, Parkinson's disease	Controversial data. Not indicated in guidelines	[36] [63]
Dexmedetomidine	Optional bolus 0.5–1 µg/kg/20 mins, then between 0.2 and 1.4 µg/kg/h dosage until desired sedation level is reached	Bradycardia, hypotension	Bradycardia, high degree AV block, caution in hypotension	Shortened duration of delirium compared with placebo in intubated patients	[52] [63] [60]
Quetiapine	12.5-100 mg bid	QTc prolongation, extrapyramidal effects	Prolonged QTc	Shortened duration of delirium compared with placebo	[81]
Olanzapine	2.5–5 mg	QTc prolongation	Prolonged QTc	Similar to haloperidol PO	[82]
Risperidone	0.5–1 mg bid			Similar to haloperidol PO	[83]

Depression is frequent in patients with heart failure (the percentages range from 15% to 60%), with an increase in the last weeks of life [2], and is an independent risk factor in reduced treatment compliance, increase of hospital admission, and mortality [89].

It is not easy to diagnose depression in patients with heart failure, as the symptoms are often masked by fatigue, anorexia, and sleep disorders, and these are not always correctly ascribed to mood disorders.

Even if there is no clear evidence of efficacy, selective serotonin reuptake inhibitors (SSRIs) are currently the first-choice drugs: sertraline (50–100 mg/day) can be used, with attention for potential hyponatremia, fluoxetine 20 mg, citalopram 10–40 mg (attention for possible QT interval prolongation), paroxetine 20–40 mg, escitalopram 5–20 mg, and mirtazapine 7.5–30 mg. Benzodiazepines are the most commonly used drugs in the treatment of anxiety, although there is insufficient data supporting their recommendation at the end of life.

The administration of psychotropic drugs should always be adapted to patient age, general clinical conditions, renal and hepatic function, and knowledge of possible side effects.

3.3.1 Fatigue

The North American Nursing Diagnosis Association (NANDA) defines fatigue as an overwhelming sustained sense of exhaustion and decreased capacity for physical and mental work at a usual level [90].

Fatigue is a common symptom in ICU (up to 70% of cases) [45] that greatly impacts patients' quality of life.

There are many causal factors: psychological (stress, anxiety, depression), physiological (sleep disorders), underlying chronic diseases, drugs—including beta-blockers, diuretics, and ACE inhibitors—malnutrition, anemia, pain, and environmental (noise, light, etc.).

Fatigue has a prevalence variable of between 60% and over 80% in heart failure patients, and is linked to higher mortality rates [90].

In advanced end-stage heart failure patients, an increased catabolic state leads to cachexia and malnutrition. In addition, nocturnal symptoms, such as paroxysmal dyspnea, orthopnea, and pain, all interfere with sleep and impact day fatigue.

The scores adopted to measure fatigue are generally validated in neurological, oncological, and infectious diseases, rarely cardiovascular. The most used fatigue assessment scale in ICU is the Numerical Rating Scale (NRS).

3.3.2 Gastrointestinal Symptoms

Patients admitted to ICU often have gastrointestinal disorders, such as nausea, vomiting, constipation, and anorexia, particularly in the advanced stages of heart failure, thus favoring the onset of cachexia.

There are multiple mechanisms at the basis of the symptoms and, particularly in patients with advanced heart failure, reduction of splanchnic blood flow and venous congestion are the main ones.

Aspirin, spironolactone, digoxin, and opioids are some of the pharmacological causes of nausea. Constipation often has multifactorial origins in patients with advanced diseases, deriving from reduced nutrition, dehydration, immobility, gastroparesis in diabetic patients, and opioid administration.

Nausea and vomiting can be associated to the final stages of uremia.

Anorexia is reported in percentages ranging from 41% to nearly 70% in patients with end-stage heart failure [91], and is often associated to dysgeusia and dysphagia.

Nausea and constipation can be measured with a 5-level numerical scale or with ESAS, where tenth place "Other" can be substituted with the assessment of nausea and constipation [92].

Treatment of nausea and constipation is illustrated in Table 3.15.

Table 3.15 Suggested drugs to treat nausea and constipation

Symptoms	Recommended therapy and Dose		Precautions for Patients
Nausea	Metoclopramide 10–20 mg po iv every 4–6 h		Drowsiness
	10–20 mg iv every 6 h		S. Extrapyramidal
			↑ QT interval
	Prometazine 25 mg po every 8 h		S. extrapyramidal
	iv/im 25–50 mg/day		Constipation. Sedation
	Proclorperazine 5–20 mg every 6 h po.		Constipation
	im/iv 10–20 every 6–8 h		S. Extrapyramidal,
	Clorpromazine 10–25 mg po every 4–6 h		Sedation,
	im 25–50 mg every 6–8 h		Confusion
	Ondansetron po 8 mg every 8–12 h		Sedation
	ev 8 mg every 6–8 h		
	Haloperidol 1.5–5 mg 2–3 times a day po		S. Extrapyramidal.
	0.5–2 mg every 8 h iv		Hepatic insufficiency. Anticholinergic action Dosage is halved for the elderly
Constipation	Senna 2–4 tablets a day in one go 24–48 mg		
	Docusate (stool softener): 1 enema a day-50–300 mg a day (tablets)		
	Senna-Docusate (8.6–50 mg) 2–4 tablets a day		

References

1. Quill TE, Abernethy AP. Generalist plus specialist palliative care - creating a more sustainable model. N Engl J Med. 2013;368:1173–5.
2. Singer AE, Meeker D, Teno JM, Lynn J, Lunney JR, Lorenz KA. Factors associated with family reports of pain, dyspnea, and depression in the last year of life. J Palliat Med. 2016;19:1066–73.
3. Bekelman DB, Rumsfeld JS, Havranek EP, Yamashita TE, Hutt E, Gottlieb SH, et al. Symptom burden, depression, and spiritual well-being: a comparison of heart failure and advanced cancer patients. J Gen Intern Med. 2009;24:592–8.
4. Mizuno A, Miyashita M, Kohno T, Tokuda Y, Fujimoto S, Nakamura M, et al. Quality indicators of palliative care for acute cardiovascular diseases. J Cardiol. 2020. [Epub ahead of print]; https://doi.org/10.1016/j.jjcc.2020.02.010.
5. Elgendy IY, Elbadawi A, Sardar P, Kolte D, Omer MA, Mahmoud AN, et al. Palliative care use in patients with acute myocardial infarction. J Am Coll Cardiol. 2020;75:113–7.
6. Crespo-Leiro MG, Metra M, Lund LH, Milicic D, Costanzo MR, Filippatos G, et al. Advanced heart failure: a position statement of the Heart Failure Association of the European Society of Cardiology. Eur J Heart Fail. 2018;20:1505–35.
7. Braun L, Grady K, Kutner JS, Adler E, Berlinger N, Boss R, et al. American Heart Association Advocacy Coordinating Committee. Palliative care and cardiovascular disease and stroke: a policy statement from the American Heart Association/American Stroke Association. Circulation. 2016;134:e198–225.
8. Barnes S, Gott M, Payne S, Parker C, Seamark D, Gariballa S, et al. Prevalence of symptoms in a community-based sample of heart failure patients. J Pain Symptom Manag. 2006;32:208–16.
9. Alpert CM, Smith MA, Hummel S, Hummel EK. Symptom burden in heart failure: assessment, impact on outcomes, and management. Heart Fail Rev. 2017;22:25–39.
10. Allen L, Stevenson LW, Grady KL, Goldstein NE, Matlock DD, Arnold RM, et al. Decision making in advanced heart failure: a scientific statement from the American Heart Association. Circulation. 2012;125:1928–52.
11. Maciver J, Ross HJ. A palliative approach for heart failure end-of-life care. Curr Opin Cardiol. 2018;33:202–7.
12. Gracely RH, McGrath P, Dubner R. Validity and sensitivity of ratio scales of sensory and affective verbal pain descriptors. Pain. 1978;5:19–29.
13. Jensen MP, Karoly P, Braver S. The measurement of clinical pain intensity: a comparison of six methods. Pain. 1986;27:117–26.
14. Scott J, Huskisson EC. Graphic representation of pain. Pain. 1976;2:175–84.
15. Mentz RJ, Hernandez AF, Stebbins A, Ezekowitz JA, Felker GM, Heizer GM, et al. Predictors of early dyspnoea relief in acute heart failure and the association with 30-day outcomes: findings from ASCEND-HF. Eur J Heart Fail. 2013;15:456–64.
16. Nekolaichuk C, Watanabe S. Edmonton Symptom Assessment System—Revised (ESAS-r) administration manual. Updated version: November 13, 2019. AHS Edmonton Zone Palliative Care Program, CH Palliative Institute & University of Alberta.
17. Puntillo K, Nelson JE, Weissman D, Curtis R, Weiss S, Frontera J, et al. Palliative care in the ICU: relief of pain, dyspnea, and thirst. Report from the IPAL-ICU Advisory Board. Intensive Care Med. 2014;40:235–48.
18. Parshall MB, Schwartzstein RM, Adams L, Banzett RB, Manning HL, Bourbeau J, et al. An official American Thoracic Society statement: update on the mechanisms, assessment, and management of dyspnea. Am J Respir Crit Care Med. 2012;185(4):435–52.
19. Nordgren LF, Sorensen S. Symptoms experienced in the last six months of life in patients with end-stage heart failure. Eur J of Cardiovasc Nurs. 2003;2:213–7.
20. Johnson M, Bland M, Gahbauer EA, Ekström M, Sinnarajah A, Mc Gill T, et al. Breathlessness in elderly adults during the last year of life sufficient to restrict activity: prevalence, pattern, and associated factors. J Am Geriatr Soc. 2016;64:73–80.

21. Nelson JE, Meier DE, Oei EJ, Nierman DM, Senzel RS, Manfredi PL, et al. Self-reported symptom experience of critically ill cancer patients receiving intensive care. Crit Care Med. 2001;29(2):277–82.
22. Nelson J, Meier DE, Litke A, Natale D, Siegel R, Morrison R. The symptom burden of chronic critical illness. Crit Care Med. 2004;32:1527–34.
23. Schmidt M, Demoule A, Polito A, Porchet R, Aboab J, Siami S, et al. Dyspnea in mechanically ventilated critically ill patients. Crit Care Med. 2011;39:2059–65.
24. Witte KK, Clark AL. Why does chronic heart failure cause breathlessness and fatigue? Prog Cardiovasc Dis. 2007;49:366–84.
25. Griffo R, Spanevello A, Temporelli PL, Faggiano P, Carone M, Magni G, et al. SUSPIRIUM Investigators: Frequent coexistence of chronic heart failure and chronic obstructive pulmonary disease in respiratory and cardiac outpatients: Evidence from SUSPIRIUM, a multicentre Italian survey. Eur J Prev Cardiol. 2017;24:567–76.
26. Faisal A, Alghamdi BJ, Ciavaglia CE, Elbehairy AF, Webb KA, Ora J, et al. Common mechanisms of dyspnea in chronic interstitial and obstructive lung disorders. Am J Respir Crit Care Med. 2016;193:299–309.
27. Wysham NG, Miriovsky BJ, Currow DC, Herndon JE 2nd, Samsa GP, Wilcock A, et al. Practical dyspnea assessment: relationship between the 0-10 numerical rating scale and the four-level categorical verbal descriptor scale of dyspnea intensity. J Pain Symptom Manag. 2015;50:480–7.
28. Mador MJ, Kufel TJ. Reproducibility of visual analog scale measurements of dyspnea in patients with chronic obstructive pulmonary disease. Am Rev Respir Dis. 1992;146:82–7.
29. Kendrick KR, Baxi SC, Smith RM. Usefulness of the modified 0-10 Borg scale in assessing the degree of dyspnea in patients with COPD and asthma. J Emerg Nurs. 2000;26(3):216–22.
30. https://mrc.ukri.org
31. Pang PS, Cleland JG, Teerlink JR, Collins SP, Lindsell CJ, Sopko G, et al. Acute Heart Failure Syndromes International Working Group—a proposal to standardize dyspnoea measurement in clinical trials of acute heart failure syndromes: the need for a uniform approach. Eur Heart J. 2008;29:816–24.
32. Campbell ML. Dyspnea. Crit Care Nurs Clin North Am. 2017;29:461–70.
33. Pisani L, Hill NS, Pacilli AMG, Polastri M, Nava S. Management of dyspnea in the terminally ill. Chest. 2018;154:925–34.
34. Barnes H, McDonald J, Smallwood N, Manser R. Opioids for the palliation of refractory breathlessness in adults with advanced disease and terminal illness. Cochrane Database Syst Rev. 2016;3:CD011008. https://doi.org/10.1002/14651858.CD011008.pub2.
35. Laerkner E, Egerod I, Olesen F, Hansen HP. A sense of agency: an ethnographic exploration of being awake during mechanical ventilation in the intensive care unit. Int J Nurs Stud. 2017;75:1–9.
36. Ely EW, Truman B, Shintani A, Thomason JW, Wheeler AP, Gordon S, et al. Monitoring sedation status over time in ICU patients: reliability and validity of the Richmond Agitation-Sedation Scale (RASS). JAMA. 2003;289:2983–91.
37. Slawnych M. Management of dyspnea at the end of life. CMAJ. 2020;192:E550. https://doi.org/10.1503/cmaj.200488.
38. Devlin JW, Skrobik Y, Gélinas C, Needham DM, Slooter AJC, Pandharipande PP, et al. Clinical practice guidelines for the prevention and management of pain, agitation/sedation, delirium, immobility, and sleep disruption in adult patients in the ICU. Crit Care Med. 2018;46:e825–73.
39. Smith AK, Stijacic Cenzer I, Knight SJ, Puntillo KA, Widera E, Williams BA, et al. The epidemiology of pain during the last two years of life. Ann Intern Med. 2010;153:563–9.
40. Goodlin SJ, Wingate S, Albert NM, Pressler SJ, Houser J, Kwon J, et al. Investigating pain in heart failure patients: the pain assessment, incidence, and nature in heart failure (PAIN-HF) study. J Card Fail. 2012;18:776–83.
41. Light-McGroary K, Goodlin SJ. The challenges of understanding and managing pain in the heart failure patient. Curr Opin Support Palliat Care. 2013;7:14–20.

42. Puntillo K, Gélinas C. Chanques. Next steps in ICU pain research. Intensive Care Med. 2017;43:1386–8.
43. Mathieson S, Lin CC, Underwood M, Eldabe S. Pregabalin and gabapentin for pain. BMJ. 2020;369:m1315. https://doi.org/10.1136/bmj.m1315.
44. Leib DE, Zimmerman CA, Knight ZA. Thirst. Curr Biol. 2016;26:R1260–5.
45. Puntillo KA, Arai S, Cohen NH, Gropper MA, Neuhaus J, Paul SM, Miaskowski C. Symptoms experienced by intensive care unit patients at high risk of dying. Crit Care Med. 2010;38:2155–60.
46. Waldréus N, Hahn RG, Jaarsma T. Thirst in heart failure: a systematic literature review. Eur J Heart Fail. 2013;15:141–9.
47. Hahn RG, van Veldhuisen DJ, Jaarsma T. Thirst trajectory and factors associated with persistent thirst in patients with heart failure. J Card Fail. 2014;20:689–95.
48. Stotts NA, Arai SR, Cooper BA, Nelson JE, Puntillo KA. Predictors of thirst in intensive care unit patients. Pain Symptom Manage. 2015;49:530–8.
49. Waldréus N, Jaarsma T, van der Wal MH, Kato NP. Development and psychometric evaluation of the Thirst Distress Scale for patients with heart failure. Eur J Cardiovasc Nurs. 2018;17:226–34.
50. Leemhuis A, Shichishima Y, Puntillo K. Palliation of thirst in intensive care unit patients: translating research into practice. Crit Care Nurse. 2019;39(5):21–8.
51. Allida SM, Shehab S, Inglis SC, Davidson PM, Hayward CS, Newton PJ. Heart lung a randomised controlled trial of chewing gum to relieve thirst in chronic heart failure (RELIEVE-CHF). Heart Lung Circ. 2020;30:516–24. https://doi.org/10.1016/j.hlc.2020.09.00.
52. Burk RS, Grap MJ, Munro CL, Schubert CM, Sessler CN. Agitation onset, frequency, and associated temporal factors in critically ill adults. Am J Crit Care. 2014;23:296–304.
53. Shehabi Y, Howe BD, Bellomo R, Arabi YM, Bailey M, Bass FE, et al. ANZICS Clinical Trials Group and the SPICE III Investigators. Early sedation with dexmedetomidine in critically ill patients. N Engl J Med. 2019;380:2506–17.
54. Mateos Gaitan R, Vicent L, Rodriguez-Queralto O, Lopez-de-Sa E, Elorriaga A, Pastor G, et al. Dexmedetomidine in medical cardiac intensive care units. Data from a multicenter prospective registry. Int J Cardiol. 2020;310:162–6.
55. Jakob SM, Ruokonen E, Grounds RM, Sarapohja T, Garratt C, Pocock SJ, et al. Dexmedetomidine vs midazolam or propofol for sedation during prolonged mechanical ventilation: two randomized controlled trials. JAMA. 2012;307:1151–60.
56. Oldham MA, Piddoubny W, Peterson R, Lee HB. Detection and management of preexisting cognitive impairment in the critical care unit. Crit Care Clin. 2017;33:441–59.
57. Zuccalà G, Pedone C, Cesari M, Onder G, Pahor M, Marzetti E, et al. The effects of cognitive impairment on mortality among hospitalized patients with heart failure. Am J Med. 2003;115:97–103.
58. Qiu C, Winblad B, Marengoni A, Klarin I, Fastbom J, Fratiglioni L. Heart failure and risk of dementia and Alzheimer disease: a population-based cohort study. Arch Intern Med. 2006;166:1003–8.
59. European Delirium Association, American Delirium Society. The DSM-5 criteria, level of arousal and delirium diagnosis: inclusiveness is safer. BMC Med. 2014;12:141.
60. Agar M, Bush SH. Delirium at the end of life. Med Clin North Am. 2020;104:491–501.
61. Falsini G, Grotti S, Porto I, Toccafondi G, Fraticelli A, Angioli P, et al. Long-term prognostic value of delirium in elderly patients with acute cardiac diseases admitted to two cardiac intensive care units: a prospective study (DELIRIUM CORDIS). Eur Heart J Acute Cardiovasc Care. 2018;7:661–70.
62. Pauley E, Lishmanov A, Schumann S, Gala GJ, van Diepen S, Katz JN. Delirium is a robust predictor of morbidity and mortality among critically ill patients treated in the cardiac intensive care unit. Am Heart J. 2015;170:79–86.
63. Naksuk N, Thongprayoon C, Park JY, Sharma S, Gaba P, Rosenbaum AN, et al. Clinical impact of delirium and antipsychotic therapy: 10-year experience from a referral coronary care unit. Eur Heart J Acute Cardiovasc Care. 2017;6:560–8.

64. Mossello E, Baroncini C, Pecorella L, Giulietti C, Chiti M, Caldi F, et al. Predictors and prognosis of delirium among older subjects in cardiac intensive care unit: focus on potentially preventable forms. Eur Heart J Acute Cardiovasc Care. 2019; https://doi.org/10.1177/2048872619882359.

65. Ibrahim K, McCarthy CP, McCarthy KJ, Brown CH, Needham DM, Januzzi JL Jr, et al. Delirium in the cardiac intensive care unit. J Am Heart Assoc. 2018;7:e008568.

66. Riker RR, Fraser GL. Delirium-Beyond the CAM-ICU. Crit Care Med. 2020;48:134–6.

67. Abdullah A, Eigbire G, Salama A, Wahab A, Awadalla M, Hoefen R, et al. Impact of delirium on patients hospitalized for myocardial infarction: a propensity score analysis of the National Inpatient Sample. Clin Cardiol. 2018 Jul;41(7):910–5.

68. Damluji AA, Forman DE, van Diepen S, Alexander KP, Page RL 2nd, Hummel SL, et al. Older adults in the cardiac intensive care unit: factoring geriatric syndromes in the management, prognosis, and process of care: a scientific statement from the American Heart Association. American Heart Association Council on Clinical Cardiology and Council on Cardiovascular and Stroke Nursing. Circulation. 2020;141:e6–e32.

69. Pisani MA, D'Ambrosio C. Sleep and delirium in adults who are critically ill: a contemporary review. Chest. 2020;157:977–84.

70. Krewulak KD, Stelfox HT, Ely EW, Fiest KM. Risk factors and outcomes among delirium subtypes in adult ICUs: a systematic review. J Crit Care. 2020;56:257–64.

71. Ely EW, Margolin R, Francis J, May L, Truman B, Dittus R, et al. Evaluation of delirium in critically ill patients: validation of the Confusion Assessment Method for the Intensive Care Unit (CAM-ICU). Crit Care Med. 2001;29:1370–9.

72. Milisen K, Braes T, Fick DM, Foreman MD. Cognitive assessment and differentiating the 3 Ds (dementia, depression, delirium). Nurs Clin North Am. 2006;41:1–22.

73. Sachdev PS, Blacker D, Blazer DG, Ganguli M, Jeste DV, Paulsen JS, et al. Classifying neuro-cognitive disorders: the DSM-5 approach. Nat Rev Neurol. 2014;10(11):634–42.

74. Inouye SK, van Dyck CH, Alessi CA, Balkin S, Siegal AP, Horwitz RI. Clarifying confusion: the confusion assessment method. A new method for detection of delirium. Ann Intern Med. 1990;113:941–8.

75. Ely EW, Inouye SK, Bernard GR, Gordon S, Francis J, May L, Truman B, et al. Delirium in mechanically ventilated patients: validity and reliability of the confusion assessment method for the intensive care unit (CAM-ICU). JAMA. 2001;286:2703–10.

76. Reznik ME, Slooter AJC. Delirium management in the ICU. Curr Treat Options Neurol. 2019;21(11):59. https://doi.org/10.1007/s11940-019-0599-5.

77. Bannon L, McGaughey J, Verghis R, Clarke M, McAuley DF, Blackwood B. The effectiveness of non-pharmacological interventions in reducing the incidence and duration of delirium in critically ill patients: a systematic review and meta-analysis. Intensive Care Med. 2019;45:1–12.

78. Wu YC, Tseng PT, Tu YK, Hsu CY, Liang CS, Yeh TC, et al. association of delirium response and safety of pharmacological interventions for the management and prevention of delirium: a network meta-analysis. JAMA Psychiat. 2019;76:526–35.

79. Burry L, Hutton B, Williamson DR, Mehta S, NKJ A, Cheng W, et al. Pharmacological interventions for the treatment of delirium in critically ill adults. Cochrane Database Syst Rev. 2019;(9):CD011749. https://doi.org/10.1002/14651858.CD011749.pub2.

80. Baumgartner L, Lam K, Lai J, Barnett M, Thompson A, Gross K, Morris A. Effectiveness of melatonin for the prevention of intensive care unit delirium. Pharmacotherapy. 2019;39:280–7.

81. Devlin JW, Roberts RJ, Fong JJ, Skrobik Y, Riker RR, Hill NS, et al. Efficacy and safety of quetiapine in critically ill patients with delirium: a prospective, multicenter, randomized, double-blind, placebo-controlled pilot study. Crit Care Med. 2010;38:419–27.

82. Skrobik YK, Bergeron N, Dumont M, Gottfried SB. Olanzapine vs. haloperidol: treating delirium in a critical care setting. Intensive Care Med. 2004;30:444–9.

83. Han CS, Kim YK. A double-blind trial of risperidone and haloperidol for the treatment of delirium. Psychosomatics. 2004;45:297–301.

84. Park Y, Bateman BT, Kim DH, Hernandez-Diaz S, Patorno E, Glynn RJ, et al. Use of haloperidol versus atypical antipsychotics and risk of in-hospital death in patients with acute myocardial infarction: cohort study. BMJ. 2018;360:k1218. https://doi.org/10.1136/bmj.k1218.

85. Akgun K, Kapo J, Siegel M. Critical care at the end of life. Semin Respir Crit Care Med. 2015;36:921–33.
86. Scragg P, Jones A, Fauvel N. Psychological problems following ICU treatment. Anaesthesia. 2001;56:9–14.
87. Davydow DS, Gifford JM, Desai SV, Bienvenu OJ, Needham DM. Depression in general intensive care unit survivors: a systematic review. Intensive Care Med. 2009;35(5):796–809.
88. Parker AM, Sricharoenchai T, Raparla S, Schneck KW, Bienvenu OJ, Needham DM. Posttraumatic stress disorder in critical illness survivors: a meta-analysis. Crit Care Med. 2015;43:1121–9.
89. Konstam V, Moser DK, De Jong MJ. Depression and anxiety in heart failure. J Card Fail. 2005;11:455–63.
90. Matthews E. Sleep disturbance and fatigue in critically ill patients. AACN Adv Crit Care. 2011;22:204–24.
91. Reintam Blaser A, Preiser JC, Fruhwald S, Wilmer A, Wernerman J, Benstoem C, et al. Gastrointestinal dysfunction in the critically ill: a systematic scoping review and research agenda proposed by the Section of Metabolism, Endocrinology and Nutrition of the European Society of Intensive Care Medicine. Crit Care. 2020;24:224. https://doi.org/10.1186/s13054-020-02889-4.
92. Alpert CM, Smith MA, Hummel S, Hummel EK. Symptom burden in heart failure: assessment, impact on outcomes, and management. Heart Fail Rev. 2017;22:25–39.

The Meanings of Prognosis: When and How to Discuss It?

4

Massimo Romanò

"Taking the patient's history is as much art as science; treatment is pastoral care as well as pharmacological rationality. Prognosis has as much to do with social science data and humanistic interpretation of lives in their social contexts as with the understanding of underlying pathophysiology and pharmacology". Arthur Kleinman [1]

4.1 Introduction

The traditional model of clinical medicine can be represented by a triangle, with diagnosis, prognosis, and therapy at its vertices (Fig. 4.1).

The etymon of the word "diagnosis" lies in the concept of "knowledge via" (clinical, instrumental, social, and environmental data), while that of the word "prognosis" relates to "knowledge before" [2].

Essentially, diagnosis identifies the disease and prognosis describes its clinical course and its final, potential outcome and "also involves insight into the current and prior aspects of the patient's health" [2].

Neither are static but, almost by definition, they evolve through time influencing therapy decisions.

In fact prognosis, in the widest sense of the Hippocratic Corpus, refers to the ability of the clinician "foreseeing and foretelling, by the side of the sick, the present, the past, and the future …. Furthermore, he will carry out the treatment best if he knows beforehand from the present symptoms what will take place later" [3].

The underlying concept is that prognosis is not just a projection into the future, identified merely with the correct use of risk scores to assess life expectancy [3]. It

M. Romanò (✉)
Organizing Committee, Postgraduate Master In Palliative Care, University of Milan, Milano, Italy
e-mail: max.romano51@gmail.com

M. Romanò (ed.), *Palliative Care in Cardiac Intensive Care Units*, https://doi.org/10.1007/978-3-030-80112-0_4

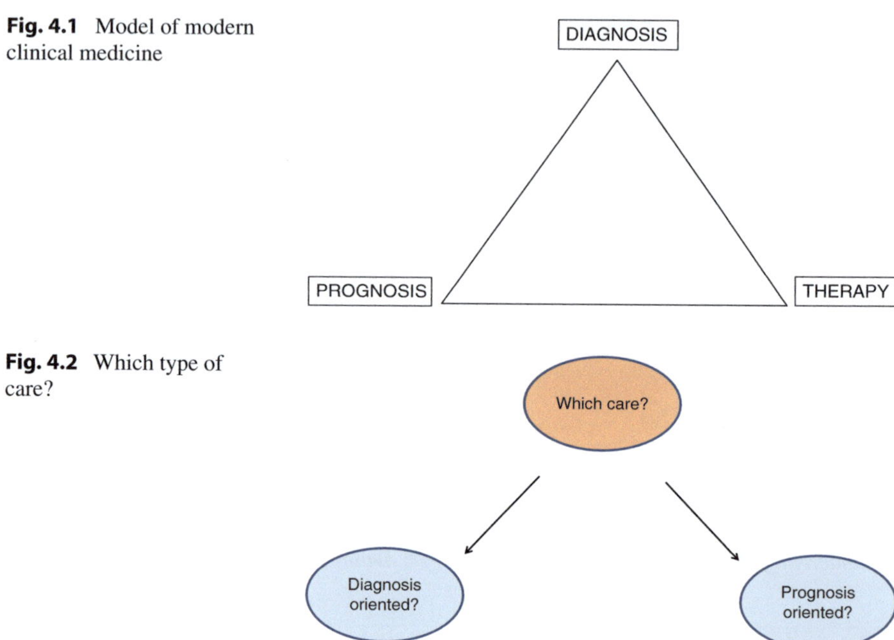

Fig. 4.1 Model of modern clinical medicine

Fig. 4.2 Which type of care?

is instead the widest knowledge of current and past aspects of the patient's health history, "so that men will confidently entrust themselves to him for treatment", with the patient being fully aware of the disease [2].

Modern medicine has changed the role of diagnosis and prognosis. The diagnosis of disease, above all in times of great knowledge advancement and particularly in the cardiological field, is at the centre of the decision-making process and care [4].

This is crucial in acute pathologies where correct and quick diagnosis allows effective therapy.

However, if applied to chronic or progressive, often relapsing diseases (for example heart failure (HF) or other pathologies that occur in modern CICUs [5]), the model does not adequately consider other important aspects concerning the complexity of the disease.

These aspects include individual variability, comorbidities, frailty, global functional assessment, social and psychological conditions, and risks connected to specific treatments, especially if invasive (Fig. 4.2).

Indeed, if we consider diagnosis-centred treatment, that can evolve qualitatively and quantitatively, we will choose care and make decisions mainly based on diagnostic and therapeutic support at high technological content. In this we are oriented by guidelines and preliminary results of precision medicine, until now applied mainly to genetic heart diseases [6] (Fig. 4.3).

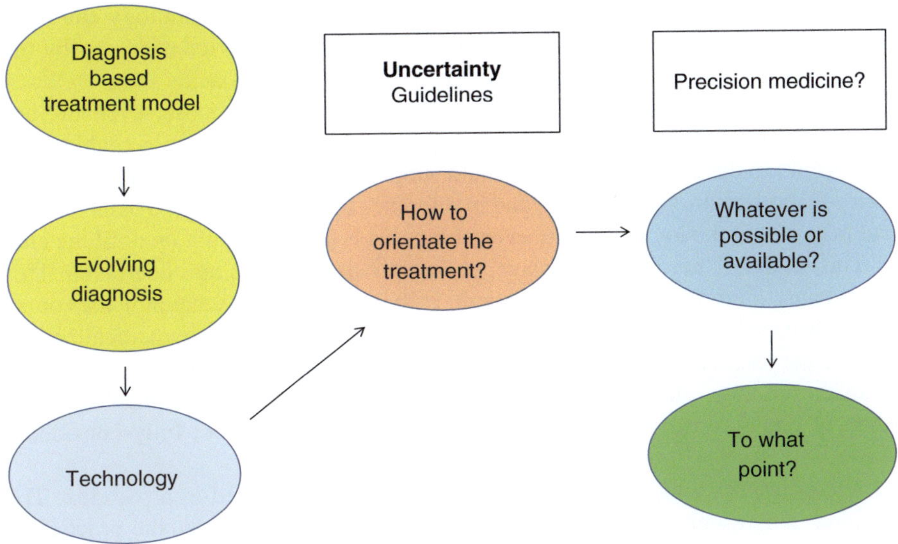

Fig. 4.3 Diagnosis based treatment model

4.2   Deciding Between Prognosis and Uncertainty

Guidelines are fundamental to clinical practice and have contributed to improving patient treatment. However, criticism of their transfer to the individual patient is well known. Individual patients eventually have different characteristics compared to the patients enrolled in the trials that the guidelines are based on. This is due to the peculiarities of patients and the areas of uncertainty that the guidelines are unable to remove [7].

The core reductionist logic prevents full assessment of the complexity of the individual patient and limits the ability of prognostic definition [8].

A recent analysis of the still valid cardiological guidelines of the American College of Cardiology/American Heart Association (with a total of 2930 recommendations) and of the European Society of Cardiology (3399 recommendations) published between 2008 and 2018 has shown that only 8.5% of the US guidelines and 14.2% of the European ones were classified with Level of Evidence (LoE) A.

This means that only a small percentage of the recommendations are supported by multiple randomised controlled trials or by single large randomised trials, but to a large extent are based on expert opinion. There is not much improvement in the 2008–2018 period compared to that of 1999–2013 [9].

So, we are often asked to manage a patient mainly using our best clinical judgment, the guidelines also being largely based on the judgement of "experts".

The diagnosis-based model contains the concepts of technological imperative and treatment imperative [9].

The overestimation in the possibilities that medicine and technology can offer and the logic of "doing everything that is possible" are supported everyday by the media. The doctor is not always able to escape from this approach.

The technological imperative refers to the tendency to choose, even in very advanced stages of the disease, some therapies just because they are available. This also occurs in the absence of documented support from controlled clinical trials on their use, both in prognostic terms and in reference to the quality of the patient's life, and falls within the logic of doing everything that is possible, right up until the end.

This leads to "heroic", aggressive, and costly therapies being undertaken. This might cause more suffering for the patient, without significantly changing the course of the disease [10], and helps disseminate the concept of infallible medical action, and the persistence of behaviour influenced by defensive medicine.

In these cases, the concept of limit, limit of reasonableness, clinical efficacy, sense of ethics, proportionality, and futility of treatment are not fully considered [11, 12].

According to Wildes, "Contemporary medicine is practiced in a paradox. The paradox is that while medicine seems to offer infinite possibilities the practice of medicine is governed by limits. No other area highlights this paradox more clearly than critical care medicine" [13].

A prognosis-centred approach, on the other hand, considers prognosis as multifactorial and can lead to a significant improvement in patient treatment, starting from a greater patient involvement in the decision-making process [4] (see Table 4.1).

The prognosis-centred care strategy, differently to a diagnosis-centred one, can include both the use of technology and the application of guidelines, even if uncertain, as they are associated to careful consideration and treatment of the patient's needs.

The patient, the disease, and its course are put at the centre of the care plan. The goal is to adopt early simultaneous treatments (disease-modifying treatments and care for the patient's needs and symptoms) and to integrate adequate technology

Table 4.1 Multifactorial prognosis assessment

- Age
- Sex
- Comorbidity
- Global functional assessment
- Pathology risk score
- Malnutrition
- Fatigue
- Frailty
- Psychological state
- Socio-economic conditions
- Lifestyle

Fig. 4.4 Prognosis-based
treatment model

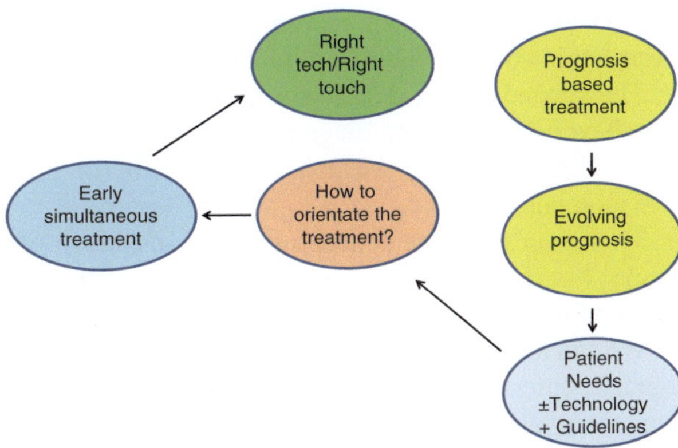

(proportional and appropriate) with the right attention to the patient's needs (right tech/right touch) (see Fig. 4.4).

At what point in the clinical processes is the intensive care cardiologist involved in key decisions concerning the critically ill patient?

When a patient with chronic disease (for example advanced HF), frail, and reduced global functional reserve is hospitalised for an acute or severe event, leading to general deterioration of clinical conditions, the cardiologist must make decisions. She/he will decide to proceed either with an aggressive therapy disease oriented or with a palliative approach and symptom-oriented treatment.

A critical aspect of this decision-making process is characterised by two fundamental factors: the first is represented by the uncertainty [14]. The second aspect deals with the concept of "the dying process".

Uncertainty concerns the diagnostic, prognostic, and therapeutic aspects.

Diagnostic and prognostic uncertainty is inherent in the practice of medicine [15]: a search on PubMed with the keywords "Uncertainty in Medicine" numbers over 17,000 bibliographic items and the more specific search "Uncertainty in Cardiology", nearly a thousand.

Sir William Osler's famous aphorism states "Medicine is a science of uncertainty and an art of probability" [16].

For many doctors, especially younger ones, it is difficult to live with uncertainty. However, physicians should accept it, understand it, and know how to manage it. Knowledge of the limits imposed by uncertainty can make clinical judgment more reliable, especially in CICU, in relation to uncertainty of prognosis in some cases and in relation to the decisions to adopt with end-of-life (EoL) patients [14].

The level of uncertainty is directly related to the degree of patient complexity, resulting from the underlying disease, the number of comorbidities, and the interactions with non-biological components (socio-familial, economic, environmental, and cultural status).

The classification of complex phenomena can be supported by models whose definition and use are referenced [17]: it is worth noting that the guidelines direct only a minority of clinical pictures, while complexity is relevant in the majority of cases but is unrepresented in clinical trials and accordingly in the guidelines.

The second aspect deals with the concept of "the dying process". This means that, beyond the specific diagnosis leading to hospital admission and to the subsequent clinical course, we are dealing with (or not) a dying patient, at a precise moment.

This process can be concentrated into a short or prolonged time, lasting days or weeks, but if initiated, it is irreversible. The unifying characteristic is the irreversibility of the clinical trajectory once it is initiated [18].

We can also intervene, with appropriate therapeutic modulation (at high technological content and/or with advanced life supports), and postpone patient death, sometimes also restoring partial cognitive and relational functions. However, we must prudently assess if our intervention will prevent death or just postpone it, if only for a short time.

The dying process is difficult to identify, as it is often masked by the global clinical picture. The diagnosis of dying should be considered in the differential diagnostic list, especially when dealing with elderly patients often admitted to CICU with multiple comorbidities and frailty [18].

In these circumstances, we are influenced by our own specific culture, professional training, religious beliefs, ethics, and prevailing values in society, including regulatory or medico-legal aspects.

This implies a discussion about the meaning of "premature death".

At what age, for which pathology, and at what stage of the disease should death be considered premature [19]?

How important is it to formulate a fatal prognosis for a critically ill patient?

This often results in withdrawing or withholding active treatments.

This prediction might influence the prognosis ("self-fulfilling prophecy") [20]: Will the patient die shortly after our decision or would they have died anyway, considering the severity of their condition [21]? It is an additional question the clinician must answer, first to herself/himself, and above all, to the conscious and aware patient and, in daily clinical practice, to the family members asking for news.

The decisions inherent to treatment limitations can be mortality markers, rather than cause of death.

However, if the "fatal" prognosis is accurately defined and empathetically communicated, also when treatment is withdrawn or withheld, the mechanism of death can change, but not its outcome.

4.3   Criteria for Prognosis Definition

Prognostic predictions are overall oriented to facilitate the timely adoption of eventual advanced treatments and/or palliative care; to choose appropriate and proportional treatments (beneficence/non-maleficence); to orient care choices towards the patient's actual needs; to promote the freedom of personal choice (autonomy); and to equally distribute the human and economic resources available (just distribution) [22].

Discussion of prognosis is difficult and challenging for the physician, the patient, and family members. It is a complex process that involves the timing of communication (during the acute or stable stage of illness), the uncertainty and unpredictability of the disease, the extent to which the patient and family members desire to know how long the patient has to live, and the quality of the remaining life [23].

The physician should clarify what actually can be done in terms of treatment, according to the patient's expectations, in the face of uncertainty [23].

The need to discuss the prognosis with patients/family members in CICU is also linked to admission criteria, which have not yet been defined and shared by Scientific Societies.

Among the main admission criteria, identified by Van Diepen et al. [24], there is the need/opportunity to use advanced treatments available in the CICU, together with the patient's specific clinical characteristics and goals of care. It is also essential to assess the nurse-to-patient ratio and the risk of clinical deterioration. Most importantly, if the prognosis is unfavourable in the short term (the patient is terminally ill) or is uncertain, then admission to CICU is inappropriate in the former case and potentially appropriate in the latter.

Two conclusions emerge.

Firstly, there is the widely shared view that low-risk patients or patients with an unfavourable prognosis which is not modifiable by CICU treatments are often admitted to CICU.

Secondly, low-risk or poor-prognosis patients admitted to CICU may undergo invasive and aggressive treatments in an inappropriate way. These can be detrimental to the quality of life and create a high level of family stress [25].

The prognostic assessment must be multi-parametric. The most relevant prognostic factors for risk assessment for death are the estimation of patient global functioning (age, nutritional state, frailty, cognitive profile, and functional autonomy) [22], comorbidities [26] (employing the Charlson Comorbidity Index), and cardiovascular system condition.

For this purpose, risk scores for predicting death such as Sequential Organ Failure Assessment (SOFA), Outcome and Assessment Information Set (OASIS), Acute Physiology and Chronic Health Evaluation (APACHE) III, and APACHE IV, which are regularly employed in ICUs, are also used in CICUs [27, 28].

Data related to risk scores for unselected patients admitted to a modern CICU is scarce [29–31].

The Mayo Clinic group has developed an in-hospital risk of death score, the Mayo CICU Admission Risk Score (M-CARS). It relies on clinical and simple laboratory variables, recorded at admission to CICU: cardiac arrest, shock, respiratory failure, Braden Scale for Predicting Pressure Sore Risk [30], urea, anion gap, and red blood cell distribution width (RDW) [29].

Noteworthy is the inclusion of a frailty measurement, the Braden Scale. This relies on a simple clinical tool, used by nurses to assess the risk of pressure-induced skin lesions. It considers patient mobility, sensorial perception, nutrition, level of hydration, friction, and shear. The Braden Scale allows assessment of the integrity of the skin and the general state of the patient.

Less clear is the meaning attributed to the RDW that indicates whether red blood cell volume is homogeneous or if there is some variability.

The physiopathological mechanism connected to the haematopoietic anomaly is not clear; it might be secondary to an increase of inflammatory cytokine secretion, oxidative stress, or neuro/hormonal activation. These are potentially related to disease severity and to a subsequent poor prognosis [30].

The same group applied another risk score, the Get With the Guidelines-Heart Failure (GWTG-HF) Risk Score, developed for patients admitted for HF, to an unselected population of patients admitted to modern CICUs.

The assumption was that the risk factors for death are similar in patients with HF or with other diseases.

GWTG-HF Risk Score showed good prognostic values even in this heterogeneous population [31].

When approaching patients with cancer or advanced chronic-degenerative diseases, evaluation of patients' needs of palliative care is done by employing the surprise question (SQ). The question, used as a screening tool, is: "Would I be surprised if this patient died in the next 12 months?" If the answer is negative, a palliative approach should be considered. If the answer is positive, the disease-modifying treatments must continue.

The SQ, designed to stimulate clinical reflection, has over time assumed the meaning of a prognostic parameter. However it is unfit for patients with non-cancer diseases, particularly those with HF, in which the specificity is only 22% with scarce positive predictive value (50%) [32]. Therefore, it should not be used as a prognostic tool.

4.4 Communicating Prognosis

Current epidemiological data [5, 28, 33] indicates that only around 30% of patients admitted to CICU suffer from acute coronary syndrome. The specific treatments and prognosis are well established [34].

Most patients, on the other hand, are affected by cardiovascular and non-cardiovascular chronic relapsing diseases [27].

In these cases there are multiple problems in prognostic definition and communication:

1. The need to trace back the previous course of the disease to know how well informed the patient and family members/caregiver are about the disease. Have the different stages of the disease, its possible evolution, the multiple treatment options, and the potential sudden and unpredictable events been discussed with their physician?
2. The identification of the patient's preferences regarding the prognostic information they wish to receive. This varies from patient to patient and in the different

phases of disease. Together with the patient, the cardiologist should further explore this issue to improve patient information and awareness and that of the family/caregiver.

3. The widest definition of prognosis does not merely include how long the patient has to live, but also the quality of the remaining life and the suffering due to the disease and due to disproportionate or inappropriate CICU therapies. Not only should the *quoad vitam* prognosis be considered, but also *quoad valetudinem*.

   Patients with serious chronic pathologies are sometimes more concerned with the fear of losing functional autonomy than from their awareness of remaining life [23].

   The last issue, not to be neglected, is the appropriateness of care location when planning complex invasive procedures.

   Hence the need to design treatment modalities based on criteria ensuring proportionality of care, which is derived from balancing the appropriateness and burdensomeness of treatments (Table 4.2) and adopting a correct bioethical approach (autonomy, beneficence, non-maleficence, justice). The proportionality of treatment must be individualised, for each particular patient, considering their clinical, social, and personal values. These must be assessed by both the physician and the patient, or the health proxy, if present and the patient is incompetent.

   These treatments are sometimes excessive and incompatible with the patient and family's wishes and expectations, and could only be the rough application of therapeutic techniques [35].

   Due to the uncertainty in prognosis, patients are unable to gain advantage from the dual contributions resulting from active treatment continuation, but also from the awareness and discussion with the care team of the possibility of death from the disease.

   It is essential to implement a shared decision-making process with the patient and family members. The goals are the assessment and therapy of physical and psychological symptoms and the discussion of shared care planning (SCP) [2].

Table 4.2 Factors affecting proportionality of treatments

Proportionality of treatments	
Appropriateness	Burdensomeness
• Suitability of care and place of care	• Costs in terms of suffering caused to the patient vs. expected benefits
• Rationale (efficacy and chances of success)	
• Durability of results	
• Financial costs	
• Complications	
• Ethics (conflict of interest)	

4. SCP enables patients to define their preferences and expectations from therapeutic options and the agreement between the treatments chosen and those received.

   It is a process that helps adult patients of any age or health condition to understand and share their personal values, life objectives, and preferences in terms of future healthcare from a physical, psychological, social, and spiritual point of view.

   Advance directives (ADs) are an essential part of SCP; ADs were defined as the presence of a living will, do-not-resuscitate order, do-not-hospitalise order, medication restriction, or feeding and hydration restriction, in the case of future loss of competence [36].

   The discussion of these aspects should start early in the course of the disease and not be left to the final stages.

   Communication on patient end-of-life choices and treatment goals, if conducted properly, does not increase patient stress, anxiety, or depression, and does not reduce hope [37].

   End-of-life conversations are associated with a better quality of life and a lower use of life-sustaining treatment near death.

   In contrast, a lack of adequate communication, or if delayed, increases patient and clinician stress, anxiety, and depression. It reduces quality of life and makes the management of family mourning more complex [38].

   Sometimes the patient and family members might disagree on the different preferences and values relating to life-sustaining treatments and cardiopulmonary resuscitation [39]. This critical situation can adversely affect SCP and ADs.
5. Patients affected by severe chronic diseases should know that acute and unpredictable clinical events could develop, even leading to death. They should be supported in preparation for these events, without reducing hope for survival and maintaining a satisfactory quality of life [23].

4.5 Barriers to Communication

4.5.1 The Disease

Overall, patients admitted to CICU present chronic, progressive, and relapsing illnesses, with comorbidities. These are clinical conditions, especially chronic organ failure, characterised by frequent recurrences, during which the patient can die, and that inevitably lead to a global, progressive decline in the quality of life. It is therefore not easy to clearly identify when the end-stage phase is approaching, consequently affecting the timing of communication between cardiologist and patient.

4.5.2 The Patient

Patient willingness to communicate is highly variable according to the specific and personal psychological context. However, this is often inseparable from the doctor's level and methods of communication, and the type of message perceived by the patient. Uncertainty generates anxiety, depression, and fear of losing hope, thus raising barriers that the cardiologist cannot overcome.

Uncertainty has an impact on all aspects of everyday life and is difficult for the patient to live with and manage [40].

Sometimes patients prefer ignoring their own clinical and prognostic situation or wish to hear only good news; in other cases, they request the truth so they can plan for the future.

However, they often complain of missing, incomplete, or misleading information [41, 42].

4.5.3　Treatment Approach

The general aims of critical CICU patient therapy are increasingly more often directed to life-sustaining treatments, while waiting for the underlying disease and/ or the acute condition to be positively resolved. In these cases, the aim is to gain time. Sometimes, however, the disease is in its terminal stage and is no longer treatable: this makes life-sustaining treatments progressively ineffective.

Moreover, the patient admitted to CICU is often submitted to therapies that could be considered futile. These aggressive and invasive treatments, at the end of life, are often excessive and incongruent with the wishes and expectations of the patient and family members.

But though Medicare patients have expressed, in over 70% of cases, the wish to receive palliative care at the end of life yet in around half of the cases death occurred in hospital and in a quarter of cases in ICU [43].

4.5.4　The Doctor

In CICU the mortality rate ranges from 5.6% to 7.4% and deaths occur in 30% of cases within the first 24 h [44].

This means that cardiologists often overestimate the effects of intensive care treatment and underestimate the risks [45]: essentially, they overestimate the prognosis, and this has been known for a long time [46].

Physician training is addressed to always fighting death, even when this is no longer feasible, and all available technologies should be used to reach this objective, independently of human, social, and economic costs.

The false perception of treatment possibilities influences communication with the patient and family members and can generate false hope, with the risk of prolonging disproportionate treatment and further patient suffering [47].

On the other hand, there is contrasting data showing that over 80% of Dutch and Swedish interviewed cardiologists are willing to discuss the prognosis with patients suffering from HF.

However, they pointed out major barriers such as lack of time, patient cognitive aspects, unpredictability of prognosis, and fear of removing patient hope [48].

Cardiologists should familiarise themselves with some subjects that are now largely unfamiliar:

(a) Living with prognostic uncertainty in a more suitable way and learning the ability to share ethical discussions within a team [49].
(b) Following a communication training programme with patients on end-of-life issues.
(c) Managing stress connected to patient discussion about death and dying.
(d) Identifying the correct timing and setting for communication.
(e) Embracing the "less is more" culture proposed by the Choosing Wisely movement, aimed at reconsidering care strategies [25], especially regarding life-sustaining treatments. Sometimes doing less can lead to more advantages for the patient: when considering disease-modifying therapies, is it always true that what is good at fighting the disease is always best for the patient [50]?

It is necessary to identify different outcomes other than survival. Also for CICU the success of intensive care treatment cannot merely be measured by survival data, but also by the quality of life preserved or restored, quality of death, and quality of human relationships involved in each death [51].

4.6 Conclusions

In most Western countries there is no formal communication training in medicine: Chap. 14 is dedicated specifically to this important issue. There are various suggestions in literature on how to solve these limits.

Regardless of the efficacy of these tools, some simple elements should be considered [52]:

1. Sharing clinical information with the patient, particularly everything related to the prognosis. It is essential to have previously shared this information within the care team.
2. Defining with the patient and family members/caregivers the goals of the treatment, the ethical and personal values at the core of the choices, and the priorities.
3. Discussing and defining the options, risks, and benefits of possible therapies, above all life-sustaining and invasive ones, and cardiopulmonary resuscitation (defibrillation, external cardiac massage, ventilation, and eventual orotracheal intubation).

According to Daniel Sulmasy [53], who discusses these problems through the analysis of a poem by Thomas Eliot, "The Love Song of J. Alfred Prufrock", everything has a meaning, but it is insufficient if we do not reflect in depth on the inevitability of death, and the uncertainty of our ethical decisions at the end of life.

The improvement of patient care at the end of life can only occur through a cultural change that brings with it the ability to fully live our lives, to face our fears (the physician's and the patient's), and to learn to live with uncertainty.

"… to emulate the virtues of the wise ones among us who are truly good persons as well as technically excellent physicians. That might be a challenge, but I am convinced that this is the key to improving care at the end of life. Eliot would ask us, do we dare?"

References

1. Kleinman A. Catastrophe and caregiving: the failure of medicine as an art. Lancet. 2008;371:22–3.
2. Thomas JM, Cooney LM Jr, Fried TR. Prognosis reconsidered in light of ancient insights-from Hippocrates to modern medicine. JAMA Intern Med. 2019;179:820–3.
3. Hippocrates. Prognostic. Translated by W. H. S. Jones. Loeb Classical Library 148. Cambridge, MA: Harvard University Press; 1923.
4. Croft P, Altman DG, Deeks JJ. The science of clinical practice: disease diagnosis or patient prognosis? Evidence about "what is likely to happen" should shape clinical practice. BMC Med. 2015;13:20.
5. Bohula EA, Katz JN, van Diepen S, Alviar CL, Baird-Zars VM, et al. Demographics, care patterns, and outcomes of patients admitted to cardiac intensive care units: the critical care cardiology trials network prospective North American Multicenter Registry of cardiac critical illness. JAMA Cardiol. 2019;4:928–35.
6. Feldman AM. Precision medicine for heart failure: back to the future. J Am Coll Cardiol. 2019;73:1185–8.
7. Lee D. Are guidelines mantra? Musings about uncertainty in medicine. J Card Fail. 2016;22:483–4.
8. Ahn AC, Tewari M, Poon CS, Phillips RS. The clinical applications of a systems approach. PLoS Med. 2006;3:e209.
9. Fanaroff AC, Califf RM, Windecker S, Smith SC Jr, Lopes RD. Levels of evidence supporting American College of Cardiology/American Heart Association and European Society of Cardiology Guidelines, 2008-2018. JAMA. 2019;321:1069–80.
10. Mueller P, Hook CC. Technological and treatment imperatives, life-sustaining technologies, and associated ethical and social challenges. Mayo Clin Proc. 2013;88:641–4.
11. Romanò M. The role of palliative care in the cardiac intensive care unit. Healthcare (Basel). 2019;7:30. https://doi.org/10.3390/healthcare7010030.
12. Schneiderman LJ, Jecker NS, Jonsen AR. The abuse of futility. Perspect Biol Med. 2018;60:295–313.
13. Wildes KW. The moral paradox of critical care medicine. In: Wildes KW, editor. Critical choises and critical care. Catholic perspective on allocating resources in intensive care medicine. Dordrecht/Boston/London: Academic Publisher; Kluwer; 1995. p. 1–4.
14. Ridley S, Fisher M. Uncertainty in the end of life care. Curr Opin Crit Care. 2013;19:642–7.
15. Kimbell B, Murray SA, Macpherson S, Boyd K. Embracing inherent uncertainty in advanced illness. BMJ. 2016;354:i3802. https://doi.org/10.1136/bmj.i3802.
16. Bean RB, Bean WB. Sir William Osler: aphorisms from his bedside teachings and writings. New York: H. Schuman; 1950.
17. Kurtz F, Snowden DJ. The new dynamics of strategy: sense-making in a complex and complicated world. IBM Syst J. 2003;3:462–83.
18. Hilton AK, Jones D, Bellomo R. Clinical review: the role of the intensivist and the rapid response team in nosocomial end-of-life care. Crit Care. 2013;17:224.
19. Callahan D. Remembering the goals of medicine. J Eval Clin Pract. 1999;5:103–6.
20. Wilkinson D. The self-fulfilling prophecy in intensive care. Theor Med Bioeth. 2009;30:401–10.
21. Sulmasy DP. Do patients die because they have DNR orders or do they have DNR orders because they are going to die? Med Care. 1999;37:719–21.

22. Romanò M. Facilitating supportive care in cardiac intensive care units. Curr Opin Support Palliat Care. 2020;14:19–24.
23. Paladino J, Lakin JR, Sanders JJ. Communication strategies for sharing prognostic information with patients: beyond survival statistics. JAMA. 2019;322:1345–6.
24. van Diepen S, Katz JN, Morrow DA. Will cardiac intensive care unit admissions warrant appropriate use criteria in the future? Circulation. 2019;140:267–9.
25. Ricou B, Piers R, Flaatten H. 'Less is more' in modern ICU: blessings and traps of treatment limitation. Intensive Care Med. 2020;46:110–2.
26. Charlson ME, Pompei P, Ales KA, MacKenzie CR. A new method of classifying prognostic comorbidity in longitudinal studies: development and validation. J Chronic Dis. 1987;40:373–83.
27. Goldfarb M, van Diepen S, Liszkowski M, Jentzer JC, Pedraza I, Cercek B. Noncardiovascular disease and critical care delivery in a contemporary cardiac and medical intensive care unit. J Intensive Care Med. 2019;34:537–43.
28. Jentzer JC, Bennett C, Wiley BM, Murphree DH, Keegan MT, Gajic O, et al. Predictive value of the sequential organ failure assessment score for mortality in a contemporary cardiac intensive care unit population. J Am Heart Assoc. 2018;7:e008169.
29. Jentzer JC, Anavekar NS, Bennett C, Murphree DH, Keegan MT, Wiley B, et al. Derivation and validation of a novel cardiac intensive care unit admission risk score for mortality. J Am Heart Assoc. 2019;8:e013675. https://doi.org/10.1161/JAHA.119.013675.
30. Jentzer JC, Anavekar NS, Brenes-Salazar JA, Wiley B, Murphree DH, Bennett C, et al. Admission Braden skin score independently predicts mortality in cardiac intensive care patients. Mayo Clin Proc. 2019;94:1994–2003.
31. Lyle M, Wan SH, Murphree D, Bennett C, Wiley BM, Barsness G, et al. Predictive value of the get with the guidelines heart failure risk score in unselected cardiac intensive care unit patients. J Am Heart Assoc. 2020;9:e012439. https://doi.org/10.1161/JAHA.119.012439.
32. Straw S, Byrom R, Gierula J, Paton MF, Koshy A, Cubbon R, et al. Predicting one-year mortality in heart failure using the 'Surprise Question': a prospective pilot study. Eur J Heart Fail. 2019;21:227–34.
33. Jentzer JC, van Diepen S, Barsness GW, Katz JN, Wiley BM, Bennett CE, et al. Changes in comorbidities, diagnoses, therapies and outcomes in a contemporary cardiac intensive care unit population. Am Heart J. 2019;215:12–9.
34. Smilowitz NR, Mahajan AM, Roe MT, Hellkamp AS, Chiswell K, Gulati M, et al. Mortality of myocardial infarction by sex, age, and obstructive coronary artery disease status in the ACTION registry-GWTG (acute coronary treatment and intervention outcomes network registry-get with the guidelines). Circ Cardiovasc Qual Outcomes. 2017;10:e003443. https://doi.org/10.1161/CIRCOUTCOMES.116.003443.
35. Dy S. Ensuring documentation of patients' preferences for life-sustaining treatment: brief update review. Agency for Healthcare Research and Quality; 2013.
36. Rietjens JAC, Sudore RL, Connolly M, van Delden JJ, Drickamer MA, Droger M, et al. Definition and recommendations for advance care planning: an international consensus supported by the European Association for Palliative Care. Lancet Oncol. 2017;18:e543–51.
37. Emanuel EJ, Fairclough DL, Wolfe P, Emanuel LL. Talking with terminally ill patients and their caregivers about death, dying, and bereavement: is it stressful? Is it helpful? Arch Intern Med. 2004;164:1999–2004.
38. Bernacki RE, Block SD, American College of Physicians High Value Care Task Force. Communication about serious illness care goals: a review and synthesis of best practices. JAMA Intern Med. 2014;174:1994–2003.
39. Abdul-Razzak A, Heyland DK, Simon J, Ghosh S, Day AG, You JJ. Patient-family agreement on values and preferences for life-sustaining treatment: results of a multicentre observational study. BMJ Support Palliat Care. 2019;9:e20. https://doi.org/10.1136/bmjspcare-2016-001284.
40. Etkind SN, Bristowe K, Bailey K, Selman LE, Murtagh FE. How does uncertainty shape patient experience in advanced illness? A secondary analysis of qualitative data. Palliat Med. 2017;31:171–80.

41. Raiten JM, Neuman M. "If I had only known". On choice and uncertainty in the ICU. N Engl J Med. 2012;367:1779–81.
42. Hjelmfors L, Sandgren A, Strömberg A, Mårtensson J, Jaarsma T, Friedrichsen M. "I was told that I would not die from heart failure": patient perceptions of prognosis communication. Appl Nurs Res. 2018;41:41–5.
43. Barnato AE, Herndon MB, Anthony DL, Gallagher PM, Skinner JS, Bynum JP, et al. Are regional variations in end-of-life care intensity explained by patient preferences? A study of the US Medicare population. Med Care. 2007;45(5):386–93.
44. Ratcliffe JA, Wilson E, Islam S, Platsman Z, Leou K, Williams G, et al. Mortality in the coronary care unit. Coron Artery Dis. 2014;25:60–5.
45. Hoffmann TC, Del Mar C. Clinicians' expectations of the benefits and harms of treatments, screening, and tests: a systematic review. JAMA Intern Med. 2017;177:407–19.
46. Christakis NA, Lamont EB. Extent and determinants of error in doctors' prognoses in terminally ill patients: prospective cohort study. BMJ. 2000;320(7233):469–72.
47. Darmon M, Benoit DD, Ostermann M. Less is more: ten reasons for considering to discontinue unproven interventions. Intensive Care Med. 2019;45:1626–8.
48. van der Wal MHL, Hjelmfors L, Strömberg A, Jaarsma T. Cardiologists' attitudes on communication about prognosis with heart failure patients. ESC Heart Fail. 2020; https://doi.org/10.1002/ehf2.12672. [Epub ahead of print].
49. Piers RD, Azoulay E, Ricou B, DeKeyser GF, Max A, et al. Inappropriate care in European ICUs: confronting views from nurses and junior and senior physicians. Chest. 2014;146:267–75.
50. Swetz K, Mansel K. Ethical issues and palliative care in the cardiovascular intensive care unit. Cardiol Clin. 2013;31:657–68.
51. Dunstan GR. Hard questions in intensive care. Anaesthesia. 1985;40:479–82.
52. Lu E, Nakagawa S. A "Three-Stage Protocol" for serious illness conversations: reframing communication in real time. Mayo Clin Proc. 2020;95:1589–93. https://doi.org/10.1016/j.mayocp.2020.02.005.
53. Sulmasy D. Advance care planning and "the love song of J. Alfred Prufrock". JAMA Intern Med. 2020;180:813–4.

Informed Consent, Advance Directives, and Shared Care Planning

5

Giuseppe Renato Gristina

5.1 Introduction

The 1995 US SUPPORT study sensitized clinicians for the first time to the issues of patient suffering and their choices [1].

Subsequently, several studies [2–11] have analyzed the issue of decision-making in the final stages of life, particularly in patients admitted to ICUs.

In the Ethicus 1 study (enrolling patients in 1999–2000), a prospective observational study involving 37 European ICUs in 17 countries, most patients (95%) were not able to make decisions and their wishes were known only in a small percentage of cases (20%) [3]. In the same study, only 1% of patients adopted ADs, decision to forgo life-sustaining treatments (DFSLT) occurred in 72.6% of patients with wide variations among European regions [3, 9], and only 14% of critically ill patients expressed informed consent.

The Ethicus 2 study referred to patients enrolled in 2015–2016 and showed a significant increase in DFSLT practice (89.7%) compared to Ethicus 1 [4].

In Australian and New Zealand ICUs only 3.2% of patients had expressed indications of some form of treatment limitation before hospital admission [7].

In 84 Italian ICUs a DFSLT was carried out on 62% of 3793 dying patients (withdrawing/withholding 34%, do-not-resuscitate—DNR—order 28%) and mainly in ICUs with a lower mortality compared to those with a higher mortality, at the same level of disease severity [5].

G. R. Gristina (✉)
Società Italiana di Anestesia Analgesia Rianimazione e Terapia Intensiva (SIAARTI)—
Comitato Etico, Rome, Italy
e-mail: geigris@fastwebnet.it

M. Romanò (ed.), *Palliative Care in Cardiac Intensive Care Units*,
https://doi.org/10.1007/978-3-030-80112-0_5

The elderly are a major issue: a multicenter Canadian study reports that 18% of patients had recorded some form of treatment limitation, and that during hospitalization another 25% had expressed such a provision [8].

Nevertheless, 72% of patients underwent mechanical ventilation and 85% received at least one of the following treatments: mechanical ventilation, vasopressor infusion, or renal replacement therapy. Forty-nine % of patients died during one of these treatments. The average time spent in ICU by patients who died was 12 days.

ADs had thus no impact on the limitation of aggressive and invasive treatments, even when family members had requested it.

In 13 French ICUs, DFSLT was recorded for 13% of patients, but during hospitalization the percentage increased to 48% of deceased patients [11].

Significant differences in the types of end-of-life (EoL) decision were recorded in line with religious beliefs and timing of activating limitations and of discussion with the patients and family members [10].

A 2011 survey showed that 66% of clinicians in Italy consider DFSLT legitimate if it respects patients' wishes [12].

However, a 2013 multicenter European survey conducted by Italian general practitioners (GPs) highlighted that out of the 2783 Italian patients enrolled in the study, affected by chronic degenerative diseases and followed up till death, only 25% had expressed a preference regarding the place of death and a mere 10% on the types of treatment, while only 5% had appointed a surrogate decision maker.

Moreover, in contrast with the rest of Europe, in Italy only 37% of patients nearing end of life turned to palliative care, whereas 90% of patients were admitted to hospitals in the last 2 months of life [13].

Other European and US studies have confirmed that not knowing patient wishes and preferences regarding therapy leads to treatment that, if the patients had been competent, they would have probably refused [14–17].

So, in Western countries, ADs have been adopted to protect patient autonomy [18].

In the USA around 70% of people who died in a nursing home, in a hospital, or at home had filled in ADs [19], but early debate has begun on their effectiveness [20] and many studies have shown that ADs modestly influence DFSLT [21] and they do not guarantee conformity between the patient's wishes and the treatment received [22–24].

A more recent systematic review of the studies published between 2011 and 2016 dealt with 795,909 cases from 150 studies. The patients had completed a living will and/or durable power of attorney for health care. The study has shown that only 36.7% of patients had completed their ADs, with little variation between people with chronic disease (38.2%) and healthy people (32.7%) [25].

As concerns ADs, there are many differences between the European countries, even in long-term-care facilities, where overall 32.4% had communicated ADs, but with a wide variability, ranging from 0 to 70% [26].

To complete this general framework there are also important notes that highlight how patients with ADs had received therapy that overall was in line with their preferences [27].

In an attempt to identify a more effective approach, the SCP model [28, 29] has been developed, in which ADs can be better integrated, and the patient can decide to accept or refuse the treatment based on the information the clinician provides.

SCP can be carried out at the beginning or during the course of a debilitating chronic disease or with a poor short-term prognosis. As with ADs, the patients can designate a health care proxy (HCP) who can decide for them while interacting with the medical team. Compared to ADs, SCP has the advantage of being developed and agreed within a patient-doctor relationship considering the specific clinical context and future evolution of disease. Consequently, in the event of patient incompetence, it is unlikely that SCP could be considered inappropriate or too general for the specific and real clinical situation.

Moreover, SCP is recorded by the doctor in the patient's electronic file so it should be easier to retrieve if the patient is admitted to ICU or general ward, something that does not occur with ADs.

5.2 Legal and Ethical Aspects

The issues of informed consent (IC), ADs, and SCP have recently acquired greater relevance both for the increasing value of patient autonomy in the clinical decision-making process and for the extraordinary progress in biomedical technology which allows long survival times. However, this is sometimes perceived as not being a real benefit by the patient, leading to disproportionate treatments.

At the same time, medical practice has largely been influenced by general greater attention to individual, civil, and political rights, and principles of social equality. This has laid the basis for the transition from medical paternalism (the doctor as the main decision maker) to patient autonomy and self-determination (patient as the main decision maker).

The requirement for IC prior to any kind of medical interventions comes from the respect for autonomy. This fundamental principle has been explicitly ratified by Article 5 of the 1997 Convention on Human Rights and Biomedicine [30].

Indeed there is now general agreement on the fundamental factors characterizing IC:

- Concerning the patient—the full mental competence; understanding of information and context; free and autonomous authorization to the medical act
- Concerning the clinician—to supply the patient, in a coercion-free context, with information suitable for their assessment of risk/benefits in that particular situation, documenting the whole information process through formal patient authorization for the treatments

Clinicians can therefore interpret IC as a three-stage process, with distinct but related phases:

- Listening—as recognition of patient rights, priorities, and preferences
- Information—as appropriate communication of technical data
- Consensus reaching—as moral choice of the patient, respecting their dignity and autonomy (the patient as moral agent)

In conclusion, IC can be interpreted from a legal and ethical point of view as a process aimed at choosing the most suitable treatment plan for the specific patient, based on clinical appropriateness and on ethical proportionality.

This approach to IC as an ethical principle that develops within the patient-doctor relationship justifies the growing interest in this respect in the Western legal tradition.

This is evident not only from the growing number of legal disputes in this domain, but also from the establishment of binding [1, 10–29, 31–33] and nonbinding [1, 20–29, 31–33] legal instruments.

Nevertheless, some circumstances facilitate the violation of patient autonomy in ICUs [34].

Organ failure, together with sedation, pain, anxiety, and delirium, alters the patient's level of consciousness, thus preventing autonomous decision-making. When dealing with critically ill patients, there is little time for extensive information to thoroughly discuss all the alternatives; family members' and HCPs' opinions may introduce uncertainty. Finally, a delay in obtaining IC increases risk for the patient [35, 36].

By contrast, critically ill patients require frequent diagnostic and invasive therapeutic procedures, with appropriate indications, which carry benefits but also some risks. Moreover, there are no specific guidelines regulating IC acquisition in ICUs.

The "implicit" consensus to treatment is still the standard approach [34, 37, 38], and patients take the risk of receiving aggressive treatment whose coherence with their preferences is effectively unclear.

When patients lose their decision-making ability, there are ethical and legal problems. In these cases it may be difficult to correctly identify a decision maker who can express consent or dissent. These same issues can arise when there is disagreement between family members and care team.

In the last 20 years, in order to ensure the respect of patient autonomy (also when incompetent) and to overcome clinical paternalism, most countries have approved laws on IC and ADs.

In 2014, the WELPICUS study defined ADs as "an instrument that relays information concerning an individual's preferences and goals regarding medical procedures and treatments, especially those used for EoL care. Advance directives intend to extend the patient's autonomy to situations in which he/she is unable to express his/her preferences regarding treatment decisions. They reflect a patient's individual moral, cultural, and religious attitudes" [39].

The WELPICUS study emphasizes that clinicians should always ask patients to complete their ADs, discussing contents with them, including ADs in the decision-making process, and certifying the patient's wishes on life support treatments, either directly or, if incompetent, with HCP or a legal representative (LR).

There might be cases in which ADs are not respected. This happens if the doctor is requested to carry out an illegal act, if there is evidence that the patient changed their treatment plan, if the ADs are not coherent with the clinical situation.

ADs can assume two different forms that are not necessarily exclusive to each other:

(a) *Living wills*: These documents are intended to allow individuals' consent or dissent to treatment, thought and written in case there is an eventual inability to make future decisions. This type of AD can be "treatment oriented" (definition of treatments that the patient declares to refuse) or "result oriented" (withdrawing or withholding treatments in case of an expected outcome or with a poor prognosis).
(b) *Lasting (or durable) power of attorney for health care*: This allows people to name an HCP to make healthcare decisions on their behalf, once they become incompetent.
(c) A combination of the two.

As previously mentioned, the theoretical ethical rationale for ADs is to guarantee respect for patient autonomy. As the patients have the right to refuse treatment, even when this is harmful to their health or may shorten their life, they should have the guarantee to continue exercising this right even when they lose their decision-making capacity.

So, other than respect for patient autonomy, it can be stated that ADs contribute to patient benefit (principle of beneficence). Indeed, thanks to ADs, patients have the right to refuse treatments they consider intolerable and unintended treatment outcomes.

Certainly, AD is based on a specific interpretation of the patient-doctor relationship that implies the right of the individual to consent to or deny consent to any treatment, including life-support tratments, even if she/he became aware of the dissent risks.

In turn, the physician must follow the patient's preferences and wishes in so far as they conform to law. This means that physicians must respect patient choice, regardless to whether they consider them clinically inappropriate.

In legal terms, since the 1990s, many Western legislation have started to regulate the efficacy and validity of ADs.

The main aspects dealt with are:

1. The methods of guaranteeing patient's full awareness of possible outcomes
2. The methods of guaranteeing that ADs are always up to date
3. Access to ADs by the physician who will take care of the patient

All legislation allow physicians a certain degree of interpretation of ADs, while respecting patient wishes.

Moreover all legal systems prefer to maintain detailed formal legal requirements to ensure the certainty of ADs.

In most cases, ADs should be archived in the patient's medical records. When a patient has not compiled their ADs, physicians must be guided by clinical appropriateness and proportionality of treatment.

It is still generally recommended to consider indications previously expressed by the patient, even if not formalized in ADs.

These principles derive not only from national law and relative Codes of Medical Ethics, but also from the application of the principles expressed in the European Convention on Human Rights (ECHR) [30], the Oviedo Convention [40], and the Charter of Fundamental Rights of the European Union (CFR) [41], and their respective legal interpretations.

The aspect that varies notably from nation to nation refers to the role and the responsibility of the designated patient representative in their relationship to the doctors.

According to the different national legal systems, different types of representatives are identified (e.g., *fiduciario* in Italy; *personne de confiance* in France; *representante* in Spain). The powers and methods of appointment vary from system to system. The shared characteristic is that HCP acts and participates in the patient-doctor relationship when the patient is not able to express their consent.

Variations on this subject include the possible existence of further representatives (legal representatives, close relatives, etc.) and of legal actions, where there is disagreement between physicians, patients, family members, or HCP [42].

In cases of incompetent patients without ADs, there can frequently be disagreement between doctors and surrogate decision makers due to differing prognostic assessments, more optimistic ones from the surrogate decision makers than those from the doctors. This leads to longer duration of life-sustaining treatments at the end of life [43].

In these situations, regular discussion of prognosis and treatment goals between clinicians and family members allows full consideration of patient values and preferences [44].

This is the standard interpretation of ADs and their underlying conceptual basis in empirical and regulatory references in the literature.

However in clinical practice, as highlighted by numerous studies, very few patients possess AD documents before their admission to ICU [34]. Also, when available, ADs do not guarantee coherence between treatments received and patient wishes [19, 45], having little influence on decisions to limit treatments [46–48], being static compared to the dynamic nature of the disease [49]. This leaves the clinician with no indications when facing other situations [50].

This may reflect situations where the patient is initially asked to supply basic information on their wish to receive advanced life supports as in the case of cardio-circulatory arrest. ADs should instead include detailed and thorough discussion involving the patient in the planning of all stages of the disease and in the preparation of choices.

Yet, despite this approach, less than 50% of involved patients complete their ADs [51].

Clinical practice and assistance in chronic degenerative diseases have identified SCP as an important opportunity to improve documentation of treatment preferences within a continuous dialogue throughout the whole duration of the disease, rather than occurring at a specific time as with ADs. ACP considers on the one hand the individual and subjective clinical progress, and on the other hand all the possible amendments that can consequently impact patient choices (wishes, preferences, and will).

SCP is thus a decisional process relying on a consultation between competent patient, clinicians, family members, and other representatives. The patient decides the level of treatment intensity/quality should she/he become incompetent. This greatly helps physicians in respecting the patient's desires [52].

SCP is a bidirectional informative process that allows healthcare professionals to know patient expectations and values, and allows patients to understand the disease severity, the prognosis, and the necessary diagnostic-therapeutic tools, while promoting informed choices and ensuring agreement between treatments chosen and those received [53, 54].

SCP models for specific clinical conditions have shown that a coordinated, systematic, patient- and family-centered approach, that includes discussions of EoL care in a shared decision-making process [55–57], improves its quality [58–60], reducing psychological stress for all people involved [61–63].

As such, ADs developed within the SCP context gain reliability and significance.

Western legislation and Scientific Societies currently support SCP models that include ADs [64–71]. The aim is to commit to improving the quality of EoL care. Still, these two tools do not seem to have achieved the expected spread among patients.

5.3 Shared Care Planning and Advance Directives in Cardiology

The survival of patients with cardiovascular diseases has significantly increased thanks to several diagnostic and therapeutic advances. However, mortality is still high, particularly in heart failure (HF) patients, and exceeds that of many cancers.

The guidelines recommend discussing ADs with patients suffering from heart disease, particularly HF [69–71]. Despite this, data supporting the prevalence of ADs in patients with severe cardiac diseases is poor.

There are several reasons to explain these data: poor training of cardiologists on discussing SCP and ADs, lack of knowledge of palliative care opportunities in HF treatment, emotional impact of SCP discussion, and absence of a multidisciplinary collaboration [72].

In order to modify clinical practice and obtain effective results in SCP implementation in heart failure [73], periodic training meetings are required. These should be offered to clinicians, family members, and patients.

Patient-family engagement programs also show a significant improvement in outcomes for CICU patients after an acute event, and the opportunity to implement SCP with the patient and to share decisions with the surrogate decision maker [74].

A more detailed study carried out in the USA has shown that the prevalence of ADs in 112 patients admitted to CICU was low and not different to that shown in a group of 105 cancer patients (26% vs. 31%). However, only 39 patients with HF and 7 with pulmonary hypertension reported to have been previously asked about ADs [75].

Subsequently, a study from Duke University analyzed a sample of 505 CICU patients [76] who were asked at admission if they had already completed ADs. 64.4% of patients ($n = 325$) did not provide ADs before hospital admission, and among the 213 patients who initially refused to complete their AD, 33.8% motivated their choice with a lack of understanding of the question.

Finally, only 48 patients completed ADs during their hospitalization.

Old age, comorbidities, and being white were directly correlated to willingness to AD. ADs were less frequent in the presence of family members, to whom the patients prevalently delegated their choices.

A Dutch observational prospective study assessed preferences in patients with severe chronic obstructive pulmonary disease (COPD) ($n = 105$) and HF ($n = 80$). Preferences were related to life-sustaining treatments, to SCP, and to communication quality on EoL issues. Patients rarely discussed ADs with their doctor (5.9% COPD patients; 3.9% HF patients), despite having the ability to indicate their life-sustaining treatment preferences based on the burden they should tolerate, on the type and probability of the outcome. Also, the majority of patients stated that in their current state of health they would have rather preferred cardiopulmonary resuscitation (CPR) (COPD 70.5%; CHF 62.5%) and/or mechanical ventilation (COPD 70.5%; CHF 66.3%) [77].

A US observational prospective study based on 608 patients affected by HF, in New York Heart Association (NYHA) class III–IV, showed that only 41% of patients had ADs at enrolment. Most ADs appointed a surrogate decision maker (90.4%), most frequently a spouse (41.8% of cases) or son/daughter (27.7%).

However patients' wishes regarding the use of EoL CPR, mechanical ventilation, and dialysis were only present in 41.4%, 38.6%, and 10.0%, respectively. Patients who had completed ADs specifying treatment limits received mechanical ventilation less frequently and fewer were admitted to ICU compared to the others, showing that ADs were not respected in all cases [78].

In another prospective study on 622 elderly HF patients (mean age 77 years) in NYHA class III–IV, EoL preferences were explored defining patient willingness to both accept a shorter life without symptoms and undergo CPR if needed.

Of the 555 respondents to the first question, 74% were unwilling to exchange survival time for a better quality of life. This percentage increased as time went on (85% after 1 year, 87% at 18 months; $p < 0.001$). Of the 603 patients that expressed their preferences regarding CPR, 51% declared accepting CPR if necessary, 39% did not want to receive CPR even if necessary, and 10% were undecided. These preferences did not correlate to final outcomes in 32% of cases [79].

A particular situation concerns patients with implantable cardioverter-defibrillators (ICD), where the device can deliver frequent and painful shocks at EoL, with no significant advantage in survival, but with a worsening of patient quality of life [80] (see Chap. 8 for details).

In these situations, it is important to decide if and how to proceed with device deactivation, in agreement with the patient or the surrogate decision maker.

However, in most cases neither the patient nor the family members are informed at ICD implantation, and in later stages of the disease, about the possibility of considering the deactivation at the EoL.

A study of 420 patients with ICD showed that 127 patients (30%) had an AD, with 83 ADs (65%) completed more than 1 year before ICD implantation and 10 (8%) completed. ADs mentioned a number of different life-sustaining treatments (artificial nutrition, 46 (37%); CPR, 25 (20%); mechanical ventilation, 22 (17%); and hemodialysis, 9 (7%)). Pain control or comfort measures were mentioned in less than 50% of ADs. However, only two ADs mentioned ICD or its deactivation at the end of life [81].

The Merchant's study is even more significant. Among 701 patients with ICDs, 23.4% had ADs, and only 1 patient made specific reference to ICD deactivation at the end of life [82].

Another study in 205 patients with cardiac pacemaker (PM) showed that 50% of patients had executed an AD (mentioning CPR, mechanical ventilation, or hemodialysis), while only 1 patient specifically mentioned possible PM deactivation at the EoL [83].

As far as do-not-resuscitate orders (DNR) are concerned, a meta-analysis conducted on 27,707 patients highlighted that DNR orders were associated with multimorbidities, above all cognitive deterioration, cancer, and stroke. The probability that a cardiac disease (coronary artery disease or congestive heart failure) was associated to a DNR was less than that for the other analyzed conditions [84].

The factors most frequently associated to the presence of ADs were analyzed in a retrospective study of 44,768 HF patients admitted to 2 US hospitals. Only 12.7% of patients possessed ADs at admission. The significant determinant factors were old age, sex (female), being white, high social-economic status, high risk of adverse outcome, expected hospital stay duration >5 days, discharge from a hospice, presence of palliative care consulting, and presence of a DNR [85].

Lastly, a Cochrane Library review assessed the effects of ACP in patients with HF compared to usual care strategies that do not have any components promoting ACP. The review included seven studies from the USA and the UK collecting data on 876 patients (mean age range 62–82; sex 53–100% male).

Only one study reported a coherence between patients' preference and EoL care, but due to the small study sample results were inconclusive [86].

Generally, there was no evidence of a difference in the quality of life between the two groups of patients. The discussions with participants could contribute to improving documentation of the ACP process.

Three studies have reported that the implementation of ACP led to a decrease of depressive burden, while there was an increase in mortality for all reasons in the ACP group.

Positive results emerge from another systematic review and meta-analysis of 14 randomized clinical trials with 2924 patients with HF: ACP improves quality of life, patient satisfaction of EoL care, and communication [58].

5.4 Conclusions

Cardiovascular diseases, especially HF and particularly in its final stages, are a unique challenge for clinicians wishing to ensure a suitable medical assistance in EoL patients, even at a human level.

The accurate prediction of the time of death in chronic heart disease patients is particularly difficult due to often-present lifesaving devices, advanced and effective pharmacological treatments prolonging life, and course of the disease, although punctuated by increasingly severe recurrences.

Nevertheless, there is solid evidence that healthcare professionals still have difficulty in communication with patients and their caregivers on EoL care preferences.

Palliative care and EoL discussions should occur before the disease trajectory approaches the final stages. Although many Western countries' legal systems have included ADs, ACP, and HCP appointment in their legislative systems, a culture of EoL choices and planning is not yet widespread.

Clinicians will understand how patients and their caregivers perceive the future only by offering them early exhaustive knowledge on future stages and possible directions of the disease. This allows clinicians to prepare patients and caregivers to identify the different disease stages and to determine if communication and discussions reduce discomfort and improve palliative care outcomes.

The advanced HF patient may represent the main model for integrating palliative care (intended in the broad sense as the treatment of all patient's physical, psychological, family, and social needs) into the experience of illness, developing the simultaneous care approach [87].

From this perspective a 2004 consensus conference identified five questions dealing with EoL assistance for CHF patients.

Even after many years [88], these questions are still pertinent today:

- How can the physical, mental, and social burdens be reduced for advanced HF patients and their families?
- Which patients receive benefits from what treatments?
- Which treatments improve quality of life, obtaining the results sought by patients and family members?

- How can you coordinate assistance between different care locations?
- Which is the best way to communicate prognosis and treatment options?

These five questions effectively summarize some of the gaps that are currently present in the discussion with terminally ill HF patients. The American Heart Association, in liaison with the Heart Failure Society of America and the American Association of Heart Failure Nurses, have issued a joint declaration on the decision-making process in advanced HF, attempting to deal with these questions [89].

Finding effective answers is still an important cultural, ethical, and social objective both for health professionals and for researchers.

References

1. The Support Investigators. A controlled trial to improve care for seriously ill hospitalized patients. The study to understand prognoses and preferences for outcomes and risks of treatments (SUPPORT). JAMA. 1995;274:1591–8.
2. Cohen S, Sprung C, Sjokvist P, Lippert A, Ricou B, Baras M, et al. Communication of end-of-life decisions in European intensive care units. Intensive Care Med. 2005;31:1215–21.
3. Sprung CL, Woodcock T, Sjokvist P, Ricou B, Bulow HH, Lippert A, et al. Reasons, considerations, difficulties and documentation of end-of-life decisions in European ICUs: the ETHICUS study. Intensive Care Med. 2008;34:271–7.
4. Sprung CL, Ricou B, Hartog CS, Maia P, Mentzelopoulos SD, Weiss M et al. Changes in end-of-life practices in European Intensive Care Units from 1999 to 2016. JAMA 2019;322:1–12.
5. Bertolini G, Boffelli S, Malacarne P, Peta M, Marchesi M, Barbisan C, et al. End-of-life decision-making and quality of ICU performance: an observational study in 84 Italian units. Intensive Care Med. 2010;36:1495–504.
6. Camhi SL, Mercado AF, Morrison RS, Du Q, Platt DM, August GI, et al. Deciding in the dark: advance directives and continuation of treatment in chronic critical illness. Crit Care Med. 2009;37:919–25.
7. Godfrey G, Pilcher D, Hilton A, Bailey M, Hodgson CL, Bellomo R. Treatment limitations at admission to intensive care units in Australia and New Zealand: prevalence, outcomes, and resource use. Crit Care Med. 2012;40:2082–9.
8. Heyland D, Cook D, Bagshaw SM, Garland A, Stelfox HT, Mehta S, et al. Canadian Critical Care Trials Group; Canadian Researchers at the End of Life Network. The very elderly admitted to ICU: a quality finish? Crit Care Med. 2015;43:1352–60.
9. Sprung CL, Cohen SL, Sjokvist P, Baras M, Bulow HH, Hovilehto S, et al. Ethicus Study Group. End-of-life practices in European intensive care units: the Ethicus study. JAMA. 2003;290:790–7.
10. Bülow HH, Sprung CL, Baras M, Carmel S, Svantesson M, Benbenishty J, et al. Are religion and religiosity important to end-of-life decisions and patient autonomy in the ICU? The Ethicatt study. Intensive Care Med. 2012;38:1126–33.
11. Lautrette A, Garrouste-Orgeas M, Bertrand PM, Goldgran-Toledano D, Jamali S, Laurent V, Outcomerea Study Group. Respective impact of no escalation of treatment, withholding and withdrawal of life-sustaining treatment on ICU patients' prognosis: a multicenter study of the Outcomerea Research Group. Intensive Care Med. 2015;41:1763–72.
12. Solarino B, Bruno F, Frati G, Dell'Erba A, Frati P. A national survey of Italian physicians' attitudes towards end-of-life decisions following the death of Eluana Englaro. Intensive Care Med. 2011;37:542–9.

13. Van den Block L, Onwuteaka-Philipsen B, Meeussen K, Donker G, Giusti F, Miccinesi G, et al. Nationwide continuous monitoring of end-of-life care via representative networks of general practitioners in Europe. BMC Fam Pract. 2013;14:73–84.
14. Winzelberg GS, Hanson LC, Tulsky JA. Beyond autonomy: diversifying end-of-life decision-making approaches to serve patients and families. J Am Geriatr Soc. 2005;53:1046–50.
15. Drazen JM, Desai NR, Green P. Fighting on. N Engl J Med. 2009;360:444–5.
16. Philippart F, Vesin A, Bruel C, Kpodji A, Durand-Gasselin B, Garcon P, et al. The ETHICA study (part I): elderly's thoughts about intensive care unit admission for life-sustaining treatments. Intensive Care Med. 2013;39:1565–73.
17. Garrouste-Orgeas M, Tabah A, Vesin A, Philippart F, Kpodji A, Bruel C, et al. The ETHICA study (part II): simulation study of determinants and variability of ICU physician decisions in patients aged 80 or over. Intensive Care Med. 2013;39:1574–83.
18. Andorno R, Gennet E, Jongsma K, Elger B. Integrating advance research directives into the European legal framework. Eur J Health Law. 2016;23:158–7.
19. Teno JM, Gruneir A, Schwartz Z, Nanda A, Wetle T. Association between advance directives and quality of end-of-life care: a national study. J Am Geriatr Soc. 2007;55:189–94.
20. Fagerlin A, Schneider CE. Enough: the failure of the living will. Hast Cent Rep. 2004;34:30–42.
21. Schneiderman LJ, Kronick R, Kaplan RM, Anderson JP, Langer RD. Effects of offering advance directives on medical treatments and costs. Ann Intern Med. 1992;117:599–606.
22. Hartog CS, Peschel I, Schwarzkopf D, Curtis JR, Westermann I, Kabisch B, et al. Are written advance directives helpful to guide end-of-life therapy in the intensive care unit? A retrospective matched-cohort study. J Crit Care. 2014;29:128–33.
23. Degenholtz HB, Rhee YJ, Arnold RM. The relationship between having a living will and dying in place. Ann Intern Med. 2004;141:113–7.
24. Potter J, Lee SW. When advance directives collide. J Gen Intern Med. 2020;35:2191–2.
25. Yadav KN, Gabler NB, Cooney E, Kent S, Kim J, Herbst N, et al. Approximately one in three us adults completes any type of advance directive for end-of-life care. Health Aff. 2017;36:1244–51.
26. Andreasen P, Finne-Soveri UH, Deliens L, Van den Block L, Payne S, Gambassi G, et al. PACE Consortium. Advance directives in European long-term care facilities: a cross-sectional survey. BMJ Support Palliat Care. 2019. https://doi.org/10.1136/bmjspcare-2018-001743.
27. Silveira MJ, Kim SY, Langa KM. Advance directives and outcomes of surrogate decision making before death. Engl J Med. 2010;362:1211–8.
28. Houben CHM, Spruit MA, Groenen MTJ, Wouters EFM, Janssen DJA. Efficacy of advance care planning: a systematic review and meta-analysis. J Am Med Dir Assoc. 2014;15:477–89.
29. Brinkman-Stoppelenburg A, Rietjens JAC, van der Heide A. The effects of advance care planning on end-of-life care: a systematic review. Palliat Med. 2014;28:1000–25.
30. Council of Europe—Convention for the protection of human rights and dignity of the human being with regard to the application of biology and medicine: convention on human rights and biomedicine https://bit.ly/2Dnr61I. Accessed June 2020.
31. Lee RY, Brumback LC, Sathitratanacheewin S, Lober WB, Modes ME, Lynch YT, et al. Association of physician orders for life-sustaining treatment with ICU admission among patients hospitalized near the end of life. JAMA. 2020;323:950–60.
32. Tyacke MH, Guttormson JL, Garnier-Villarreal M, Schroeter K, Peltier W. Advance directives and intensity of care delivered to hospitalized older adults at the end-of-life. Heart Lung. 2020;49:123–31.
33. Goodman MD, Tarnoff M, Slotman GJ. Effect of advance directives on the management of elderly critically ill patients. Crit Care Med. 1998;26:701–4.
34. Banja J, Sumler M. Overriding advance directives: a 20-year legal and ethical overview. J Healthc Risk Manag. 2019;39:11–8.
35. Fan E, Shahid S, Kondreddi VP, Bienvenu OJ, Mendez-Tellez PA, Pronovost PJ, et al. Informed consent in the critically ill: a two-step approach incorporating delirium screening. Crit Care Med. 2008;36:94–9.

36. Azoulay E, Pochard F, Chevret S, Adrie C, Annane D, Bleichner G. Half the family members of intensive care unit patients do not want to share in the decision-making process: a study in 78 French intensive care units. Crit Care Med. 2004;32:1832–8.
37. Gristina GR, Piccinni M. Informed consent in Italian intensive care units: a moral tenet or just a formal legal requirement? Minerva Anestesiol. 2013;79:708–10.
38. Kellum JA, White DB. Ethics in the intensive care unit: informed consent; 2018. http://bit.ly/2FQR4Xs. Accessed June 2020.
39. Sprung CL, Truog RD, Curtis JR, Joynt GM, Baras M, Michalsen A, et al. Seeking worldwide professional consensus on the principles of end-of-life Care for the critically ill. The consensus for worldwide end-of-life practice for patients in intensive care units (WELPICUS) study. Am J Respir Crit Care Med. 2014;190:855–66.
40. Convention on Human Rights and Biomedicine (Oviedo Convention) 1997 art. 5. https://bit.ly/2F2QxWM. Accessed June 2020.
41. Charter of Fundamental Rights of the European Union 2007 art. 3. https://bit.ly/3h1UJDO. Accessed June 2020.
42. Gristina GR, Busatta L, Piccinni M. The Italian law on informed consent and advance directives: its impact on intensive care units and the European legal framework. Minerva Anestesiol. 2019;85:401–11.
43. White DB, Carson S, Anderson W, Steingrub J, Bird G, Curtis JR, et al. A multicenter study of the causes and consequences of optimistic expectations about prognosis by surrogate decision-makers in ICUs. Crit Care Med. 2019;47:1184–93.
44. Scheunemann LP, Ernecoff NC, Buddadhumaruk P, Carson SS, Hough CL, Curtis JR, et al. Clinician-family communication about patients' values and preferences in intensive care units. JAMA Intern Med. 2019;179:676–84.
45. Wendler D, Rid A. Systematic review: the effect on surrogates of making treatment decisions for others. Ann Intern Med. 2011;154:336–46.
46. Hickman SE, Hammes BJ, Moss AH, Tolle SW. Hope for the future: achieving the original intent of advance directives. Hastings Cent Rep 2005;Spec No:S26–S30.
47. Qureshi AI, Chaudhry SA, Connelly B, Abott E, Janjua T, Kim SH, et al. Impact of advanced healthcare directives on treatment decisions by physicians in patients with acute stroke. Crit Care Med. 2013;41:1468–75.
48. Hinders D. Advance directives: limitations to completion. Am J Hosp Palliat Care. 2012;29:286–9.
49. White DB, Arnold RM. The evolution of advance directives. JAMA. 2011;306:1485–6.
50. Degenholtz HB, Rhee Y, Arnold RM. Brief communication: the relationship between having a living will and dying in place. Ann Intern Med. 2004;141:113–7.
51. National Consensus Project for Quality Palliative Care. Clinical practice guidelines for quality palliative care. 3rd ed. Pittsburgh, PA: National Coalition for Hospice & Palliative Care. Available at: https://bit.ly/2DvKrhh. Accessed June 2020.
52. Singer P, Robertson G, Roy D. Bioethics for clinicians: 6. Advance care planning. CMAJ. 1996;155:1689–92.
53. Rietjens JA, Sudore RL, Connolly M, et al. Definition and recommendations for advance care planning: an international consensus supported by the European Association for Palliative Care. Lancet Oncol. 2017;18:e543–51.
54. Sobanski P, Alt-Epping B, Currow D, et al. Palliative care for people living with heart failure: European Association for Palliative Care Task Force expert position statement. Cardiovasc Res. 2020;116:12–27.
55. Curtis JR, White DB. Practical guidance for evidence-based ICU family conferences. Chest. 2008;4:835–43.
56. Scheunemann LP, McDevitt M, Carson SS, Hanson LC. Randomized, controlled trials of interventions to improve communication in intensive care: a systematic review. Chest. 2011;139:543–54.
57. Hinkle LJ, Bosslet GT, Torke AM. Factors associated with family satisfaction with end-of-life care in the ICU: a systematic review. Chest. 2015;147:82–93.

58. Schichtel M, Wee B, Perera R, Onakpoya I. The effect of advance care planning on heart failure: a systematic review and meta-analysis. J Gen Intern Med. 2020;35:874–84.
59. Romer AL, Hammes BJ. Communication, trust, and making choices: advance care planning four years on. J Palliat Med. 2004;7:335–40.
60. Briggs L. Shifting the focus of advance care planning: using an in-depth interview to build and strengthen relationships. J Palliat Med. 2004;7:341–9.
61. Azoulay E, Pochard F, Kentish-Barnes N, Chevret S, Aboab J, Adrie C, et al. Risk of post-traumatic stress symptoms in family members of intensive care unit patients. Am J Respir Crit Care Med. 2005;171:987–94.
62. Wright AA, Zhang B, Ray A, Mack JW, Trice E, Balboni T, et al. Associations between end-of-life discussions, patient mental health, medical care near death, and caregiver bereavement adjustment. JAMA. 2008;300:1665–73.
63. Kentish-Barnes N, Chaize M, Seegers V, Legriel S, Cariou A, Jaber S, et al. Complicated grief after death of a relative in the intensive care unit. Eur Respir J. 2015;45:1341–52.
64. British Medical Association. bma-advance-care-plan-patient-information-leaflet-june-2020.pdf. www.bma.org.uk. Accessed Sep 2020.
65. Cartwright CM, Parker MH. Advance care planning and end-of-life decision making. Aust Fam Physician. 2004;33:815–9.
66. Cartwright CM, White BP, Willmott L, Williams G, Parker MH. Palliative care and other physicians' knowledge, attitudes and practice relating to the law on withholding/withdrawing life-sustaining treatment: Survey results. Palliat Med. 2016;30:171–9.
67. American Medical Association. Code of medical ethics: caring for patients at the end of life. https://www.ama-assn.org/delivering-care/ethics/code-medical-ethics-caring-patients-end-life. (ultimo accesso settembre 2020).
68. Australian Medical Association. Position statement on end of life care and advance care planning 2014. https://ama.com.au/system/tdf/documents/AMA_position_statement_on_end_of_life_care_and_advance_care_planning_2014.pdf?file=1&type=node&id=40573 (ultimo accesso settembre 2014).
69. Yancy CW, Jessup M, Bozkurt B, Butler J, Casey DE Jr, Drazner MH, et al. 2013 ACCF/AHA guideline for the management of heart failure: a report of the American College of Cardiology Foundation/American Heart Association Task Force on Practice Guidelines. J Am Coll Cardiol. 2013;62:e147–239.
70. Lindenfeld J, Albert NM, Boehmer JP, Collins SP, Ezekowitz JA, Givertz MM, et al. HFSA 2010 comprehensive heart failure practice guideline. J Card Fail. 2010;16:e1–194.
71. Crespo-Leiro MG, Metra M, Lund LH, Milicic D, Costanzo MR, et al. Advanced heart failure: a position statement of the Heart Failure Association of the European Society of Cardiology. Eur J Heart Fail. 2018;20:1505–35.
72. Schichtel M, Wee B, MacArtney JI, et al Clinician barriers and facilitators to heart failure advance care plans: a systematic literature review and qualitative evidence synthesis. BMJ Support Palliat Care. Published Online First: 22 July 2019. https://doi.org/10.1136/bmjspcare-2018-001747
73. Schichtel M, Wee B, Perera R, Onakpoya I, Albury C, Barber S. Clinician-targeted interventions to improve advance care planning in heart failure: a systematic review and meta-analysis. Heart. 2019;105:1316–24.
74. Goldfarb M, Bibas L, Burns K. Patient and family engagement in care in the cardiac intensive care unit. Can J Cardiol. 2020;36:1032–40.
75. Kirkpatrick JN, Guger CJ, Arnsdorf MF, Fedson SE. Advance directives in the cardiac care unit. Am Heart J. 2007;154:477–81.
76. Johnson RW, Zhao Y, Newby LK, Granger CB, Granger BB. Reasons for noncompletion of advance directives in a cardiac intensive care unit. Am J Crit Care. 2012;21:311–20.
77. Janssen DJA, Spruit MA, Schols JMGA, Wouters EFM. A call for high-quality advance care planning in outpatients with severe COPD or chronic heart failure. Chest. 2011;139:1081–8.
78. Dunlay SM, Keith M, Swetz KM, Mueller PS, Roger VL. Advance directives in community patients with heart failure. Circ Cardiovasc Qual Outcomes. 2012;5:283–9.

79. Brunner-La Rocca HP, Rickenbacher P, Muzzarelli S, Schindler R, Maeder MT, Jeker U, et al; for the TIME-CHF Investigators. End-of-life preferences of elderly patients with chronic heart failure. Eur Heart J 2012; 33: 752–759.

80. Kinch Westerdahl A, Sjöblom J, Mattiasson AC, Rosenqvist M, Frykman V. Implantable cardioverter-defibrillator therapy before death. High risk for painful shocks at end of life. Circulation. 2014;129:422–9.

81. Tajouri TH, Ottenberg AL, Hayes DL, Mueller PS. The use of advance directives among patients with implantable cardioverter defibrillators. Pacing Clin Electrophysiol. 2012;35(5):567–73.

82. Merchant F, Binney Z, Patel A, Li J, Peddareddy LP, El-Chami MF, Leon AR, Quest T. Prevalence, predictors, and outcomes of advance directives in implantable cardioverter-defibrillator recipients. Heart Rhythm. 2017;14:830–6.

83. Pasalic D, Tajouri TH, Ottenberg AL, Mueller PS. The prevalence and contents of advance directives in patients with pacemakers. Pacing Clin Electrophysiol. 2014;37:473–80.

84. De Decker L, Annweiler C, Launay C, Fantino B, Beauchet O. Do not resuscitate orders and aging: impact of multimorbidity on the decision-making process. J Nutr Health Aging. 2014;18(3):330–5.

85. Butler J, Binney Z, Kalogeropoulos A, Owen M, Clevenger C, Gunter D, et al. Advance directives among hospitalized patients with heart failure. J Am Coll Cardiol HF. 2015;3:112–21.

86. Nishikawa Y, Hiroyama N, Fukahori H, Ota E, Mizuno A, Miyashita M, et al. Advance care planning for adults with heart failure. Cochrane Database Syst Rev. 2020;(2):CD013022. https://doi.org/10.1002/14651858.CD013022.pub2.

87. Kavalieratos D, Gelfman LP, Tycon LE, Riegel B, Bekelman DB, Ikejiani DZ, et al. Palliative care in heart failure: rationale, evidence, and future priorities. J Am Coll Cardiol. 2017;70:1919–30.

88. Goodlin SJ, Hauptman PJ, Arnold R, et al. Consensus statement: palliative and supportive care in advanced heart failure. J Card Fail. 2004;10:200–9.

89. Allen LA, Stevenson LW, Grady KL, Goldstein NE, Matlock DD, Arnold RM, et al. American Heart Association; Council on Quality of Care and Outcomes Research; Council on Cardiovascular Nursing; Council on Clinical Cardiology; Council on Cardiovascular Radiology and Intervention; Council on Cardiovascular Surgery and Anesthesia. Decision making in advanced heart failure: a scientific statement from the American Heart Association Circulation 2012;125:1928–1952.

Withholding or Withdrawing Life-Sustaining Treatments

6

Giuseppe Renato Gristina

6.1 Introduction

In Western countries over the last decades, thanks to the advances in medical technology and pharmacology, there has been a continuous development of intensive care medicine resulting in an increasing number of general intensive care units (ICUs) and specialized ones (i.e., cardiac intensive care unit—CICU).

In 2012, the total number of ICU beds in Europe was on average 11.5/100,000 inhabitants, indicating a positive correlation with gross domestic product in each country [1].

The broad diffusion of ICUs has resulted in a continuously increasing number of hospitalized patients, while the mortality rate for acute severe diseases has reduced to the current 16% [2].

At the same time the demographic and the epidemiological characteristics of patients admitted to CICUs have greatly changed [3]. This leads to a wider variety of conditions being currently managed in CICUs, ranging from the need of cardiac monitoring to the treatment of severe cardiovascular diseases with multiple-organ failures [4–6].

In addition, there is an increasing awareness among ICU doctors that not all patients can benefit from intensive care and many should be accompanied towards a dignified death [7–10]. In these cases, treatments do not improve prognosis, but transform death into a process whose duration is proportional to the treatment intensity. This *real-life* experience has contributed to change the perception of intensive medicine among most healthcare professionals.

G. R. Gristina (✉)
Società Italiana di Anestesia Analgesia Rianimazione e Terapia Intensiva (SIAARTI)—
Comitato Etico, Rome, Italy
e-mail: geigris@fastwebnet.it

M. Romanò (ed.), *Palliative Care in Cardiac Intensive Care Units*,
https://doi.org/10.1007/978-3-030-80112-0_6

As there is no data in literature specific to CICUs, these considerations derive from ICUs' experience.

A 2007 study, on 1899 healthcare professionals, showed that most of them considered quality of life more important than the value of life itself. Moreover, if affected by a terminal disease, clinicians and nurses would have preferred entering a palliative care program rather than an intensive one [11].

Thus, most deaths in ICUs today follow a decision to limit life-sustaining treatments—decision to forgo life-sustaining treatments—DFLSTs [12, 13].

In 2015 a consensus conference [14] established the definitions of end-of-life (EoL) practices:

- Life-sustaining treatments (LSTs) are defined as those commonly considered as lifesaving: cardiopulmonary resuscitation, mechanical ventilation with or without endotracheal intubation, mechanical circulatory supports or cardiac electronic devices, use of vasopressors and/or cardioactive drugs, renal replacement therapies, artificial nutrition, and massive use of blood products, antibiotics, and intravenous fluids.
- If LSTs cannot improve prognosis but only prolong the dying process, clinicians should refrain from using them, discussing this choice with the patient if possible, or with their healthcare proxy if present, or with family members.
- LSTs must be used according to the patient's preferences and values. If a patient does not want to start or continue a LST and this desire is expressed in full awareness or in the ways provided by law, this must be respected.
- DFLSTs can be performed in two ways: withholding life-sustaining treatments (WHLST) or withdrawing life-sustaining treatments (WDLST). WHLST can refer to the decision not to start LSTs (for example not practicing cardiopulmonary resuscitation in the event of a cardiocirculatory arrest—do not resuscitate, DNR), or the decision not to intensify the ongoing LSTs, if the disease worsens or with the onset of particular complications (do not escalate, DNE) [15].
- The active shortening of the dying process (ASDP) is defined as the circumstance in which the physician takes action in order to shorten the dying process of the patient. This links to the definition of euthanasia and should not be confused with WHLST or WDLST.

6.2 Forgoing Life-Sustaining Treatments: The Clinical Practice

A wide variability regarding the two methods of carrying out a DFLST has been reported between different geographic areas, ICUs, and intensive care groups [16].

As suggested by numerous studies, several factors are associated with the significant differences in the prevalence of one DFLST method to another. These include the clinician's cultural background, their religious affiliation, and various legislative frameworks [17].

ICUs in Eastern countries and Israel report a major prevalence of WHLST practice [18–21] whereas in Western countries more recourse to WDLST seems to be increasing over time [22], being influenced by factors such as availability of a trustee [23], patient's advanced age [24], and severe, irreversible disease [25].

These factors account for only one part of the variability.

Three studies carried out in ICUs in England [26], the USA [27], and Europe [5] have shown a wide range of WDLST prevalence (0–96%, 0–79%, and 5–69%, respectively).

The same result arose in another US study, carried out in 153 ICUs. The study considered the relationship between the patients' demographic and social characteristics, the type and severity of the disease, and the ICUs' organizational models [28].

In an additional US study, only 34% of 1446 healthcare professionals considered WHLST and WDLST as equivalent [26].

Another study conducted in Italy in 2003 explored the perception regarding DFLST of 225 clinicians across 20 ICUs in Milan (Lombardy region). Seventy-seven % of clinicians considered the proportion of deaths preceded by DFLST ranging from 1 to 10% of cases, while 53% affirmed that there was no ethical difference between WHLST and WDLST.

Twenty-six % considered WHLST morally more acceptable than WDLST. On the other hand, 51% of clinicians judged WDLST as psychologically more complex and strenuous to deal with, compared to WHLST. The main reasons for the DFLST were identified as the lack of response to full treatment (42%), the futility of treatment (50%), the severity of the underlying disease (48%), or a preexisting neurological disease (43%) [29].

In 2010, a study conducted on 84 Italian general ICUs showed that DFLST preceded 62% of the 3793 total deaths. In 28% WHLST was carried out via DNR, ensuring full support for the remaining treatments; in 16% of the remaining cases WHLST was practiced via DNE, while WDLST was practiced in 17%.

A particularly interesting aspect highlighted by this study concerns the higher mortality, for the same disease severity, evidenced in the ICUs with a lower-than-average propensity for DFLST. On the other hand, there was a lower mortality in ICUs with a higher-than-average propensity to DFLST indicating that DFLST was not carried out against patients' best interests [30].

Even though a systematic review of the guidelines and recommendations has shown that in 97% of analyzed documents WHLST and WDLST were considered ethically and legally equal [31] and that there is also significant agreement among physicians [32], this subject remains controversial in clinical practice.

6.3 Physician Preferences

In terms of clinical ethics, physicians seem to lean mainly for the theory of *non-equivalence*: if in some situations it is allowed not to start a treatment, it cannot be allowed to suspend one that has already started [33].

A first possible reason for this preference is that during the decision-making process the physicians tend not to modify the state of things [34]. This *status quo* bias leads physicians to judge harmful actions as worse than equally harmful omissions [35].

Therefore, they intuitively consider active treatment withdrawing worse than withholding it [36].

Regarding the relationship between WHLST, WDLST, and distributive justice, it is well known that clinicians work on a "first-come-first-serve" rule [37, 38]. This rule is simple to apply and clear. However, this leads to ethically questionable conclusions: if patient X has only 1% possibility of survival with intensive care treatment and patient Y has 99% possibility of survival with the same treatment, the "first-come-first serve" rule would give priority to X if they arrive first. A further concern, relating to WDLST practice in a context of limited resources, deals with WDLST based on morally unjustifiable criteria (ethnicity, skin color, religion, etc.). However, also with WHLST it is possible to take decisions that might prove unjust.

Another reason clinicians prefer to manage treatment limitation via WHLST is that the decision not to admit the patient to ICU can be communicated directly to the physicians requesting it from wards or emergency department, and not discussed with the patient, trustee, or family members.

In contrast, the process that leads to the WDLST decision requires previous discussion within the healthcare team, and then agreement with the patient, family members, or legal representative. However, it is always difficult to communicate to family members that continuing intensive treatment is no longer in the patient's best interests and that the healthcare team has decided on WDLST [26, 27].

As far as the legal aspects regarding WDLST/WHLST are concerned, it is necessary to highlight the perception that physicians have of their professional responsibility regarding WDLST.

In the USA, Canada, New Zealand, and some European countries including Italy, the principle of proportionality of treatment, including in the final stages of life, and resort to DFLST are all covered by specific laws. The contents of these laws vary from system to system according to the relationship with the recipients, clinical conditions justifying the procedure, methods of intervention, and clinician involvement [39].

Despite this, given the close causal and temporal relationship between WDLST and death, the physicians may fear legal disputes when involved in WDLST rather than in WHLST [26, 40].

6.4 Withdrawing Life-Sustaining Treatment: Arguments in Favor

In clinical practice, the choice for WDLST compared to WHLST would offer the patient a trial of an intensive care treatment that is interrupted if the sought-after results are not achieved (ICU test).

The ICU test may be carried out in different ways:

- **Time-limited** (maximal medical therapy over a limited time, at the end of which there may be more elements to come to a decision)

- **Event-limited** (continue the ongoing treatment but suspending it if new acute events appear)
- **Skill-limited** (continue the ongoing treatment without increasing its level)

This approach guarantees the patient a chance and the clinicians the possibility to make a prognosis based on fact, rather than remaining in the uncertainty of having denied a chance on the basis of a probabilistic calculation, albeit accurate. This argument makes a relevant difference between the two DFLST methods.

There is also another reason for which treatment interruption should be allowed.

When intensive treatment is continued despite a poor prognosis, this treatment could be denied to other patients more likely to benefit from it. This is not only a theoretical problem. Studies focusing on the ICU admission issue have also shown an increase in risk of death in patients that were refused admission, equal to 2.5 times the risk calculated after adjustment for disease severity markers [41].

6.5 Withholding Life-Sustaining Treatment: Arguments in Favor

An argument used in favor of WDLST is the usefulness of an ICU test. As a consequence of recent demographic and epidemiological changes in the Western population, the number of "end-stage" chronic patients admitted to hospital and inappropriately admitted to ICU has progressively increased. In this context, it seems that the ICU test has not reached its expected goal. A series of studies show that, once admitted to ICU, these patients undergo prolonged hospital stay with a significantly higher mortality than the average, both in ICU and within 1 year after discharge [42]. Variables such as age [43], comorbidities [44], functional-cognitive status [45], frailty [46], and quality of life before and after hospitalization [47, 48] should be taken carefully into consideration [49] for an appropriate triage [50] and when discussing with patients and their loved ones on the feasible treatment goals [51].

However, in a high percentage of cases, patients passing the ICU test are then readmitted to ICU due to subsequent clinical worsening caused by disease relapse. Readmission allows additional survival time, but ever shorter, with an increase in suffering both for the patients and their family, and in costs for the society [52].

6.6 Withdrawing or Withholding Life-Sustaining Treatments: Means or Goals?

At a theoretical level it can be agreed that there are no substantial differences between WDLST and WHLST. In both cases the decision refers to a situation where clinicians recognize that LSTs do not improve the prognosis, prolonging the dying process that leads, in turn, to more suffering for the patients and their loved ones.

The situation is different at a practical level. Differences can be better understood if two representative situations are considered.

A patient affected by a chronic-degenerative disease experiences a clinical worsening suggesting a need for intensive care. If this is disproportionate according to a clinical assessment, and WHLST is decided, the patient will not be admitted to ICU. However, it will be possible to continue ongoing treatments, while receiving simultaneous palliative care that improves the quality of the end of life and provides a dignified death in a time variable of hours to days. In contrast, if the patient is admitted for an ICU test and this does not positively modify the prognosis, deciding for WDLST means interrupting the life-sustaining treatments and starting palliative sedation. Death will follow shortly.

Some difference certainly exists between these two circumstances, regarding different types of stress, suffering, and commitment for the patient, the family members, and the whole healthcare team [53].

In light of the principle of autonomy, this difference represents an important core of information that should be passed on to the patient and family members in order to bring about a course of action in line with their preferences and values.

In conclusion, in clinical practice there is no theoretical algorithm defining which is the best or worst method for implementing a DFLST.

The only way to deal with the difficult task of caring for a patient at the end of life and communicating with family members is to adequately choose which option—WDLST or WHLST—is the best method according to patient's values and preferences and according to an overall assessment of the patient's clinical conditions and care setting (ward, ICU, emergency room).

It is then important that any decision is taken as early as possible. All possibilities should always be discussed, first within the healthcare team and then with the family members. The final decisions should be explicit, properly shared and communicated, having achieved a consensus, and finally documented on medical records.

If this is true in the case of WDLST in ICU, it is even truer in the case of WHLST outside of the ICU. This will allow everyone to deal with the approaching death in the best possible way.

6.7 Forgoing Life-Sustaining Treatments: How to Do

6.7.1 Ethical Principles

A treatment may be defined as potentially inappropriate (*futile*) if the patient is unlikely to benefit from it or, when notwithstanding a possible benefit, it is deemed inappropriate for the patient given the severity of their clinical condition [54, 55].

A treatment is proportionate, therefore legitimate and ethically lawful, only if beyond being clinically appropriate, it is also accepted with full awareness by the patient.

If the patient is no longer competent, the treatment will coherently adhere to the individual's life project, as far as it is possible to reconstruct it.

Clinical appropriateness responds to the reasonable probability that a specific treatment on a specific person can meet the sought-after beneficial expectations, positively changing the prognosis and predicting a reasonable recovery perspective.

Patient acceptance responds, however, to their personal assessment of the quality of the possible recovery. This is defined by the relationship between psychophysical benefit and burden derived from that treatment, even if clinically appropriate.

Any treatment, whether clinically inappropriate or appropriate, but not accepted by the patient and so disproportionate, must be suspended or not initiated, and this must be done in a way that respects patient dignity and family sensitivity.

In emergency cases, where it is not possible to obtain informed consent (IC) from the patient, and/or advance directives (ADs) are not available and/or clinical elements to formulate a reasonable prognosis are insufficient, the clinician proceeds to the appropriate intensive treatments. The assessment of correct treatment progression (proportionality assessment) is postponed to a later stage.

When the patient is incapable of giving IC, the clinician will refer to the ADs or the healthcare proxy or the legal guardian where present.

Without all these conditions the physician will try to reconstruct the patient's wishes through the testimony of family members, guided by the criterion of the patient's best interest [45, 46].

6.7.2 Decision to Forgo Life-Sustaining Treatments: Theoretical Approach

Clinical ethical reasoning aims at planning the best possible course of action for a specific patient. When the decision is to limit treatment (WDLST or WHLST), it is necessary to clearly distinguish and define:

1. The clinical picture (diagnosis, prognosis, possible therapeutic strategies, level and reasons of uncertainty)
2. The responsibilities (people involved in the decision-making process, healthcare team and others, and their roles)
3. The values (identification of the possible ethical dilemmas, the discordant perspectives, the potential conflicts)
4. The decision (identification of appropriate strategy, its argumentation, alternative choices)

EoL management is often difficult. Continuous, productive discussion supported by expert teamwork and shared agreement ensures quality of the method, even if there is not always unanimity on the subject.

Each department should define a protocol providing the guidelines to deal with both the decision-making process, leading to eventual treatment limitations, and any conflict of opinions within the healthcare team and/or between clinicians and family members.

If the decision to limit treatment does not meet the family members' consensus or leads to conflict, the clinician must gradually involve the family members leading them to understand and share the motivations underlying the medical decision and strategy.

This goal should be achieved without the family members carrying the moral weight of the decision.

Although good communication often leads to shared choices, sometimes it can be difficult to get family members to understand that treatment limitations represent the patient's best interest.

In this situation, expert external interventions (consultants or ethics committees) will help with conflict mediation and resolution.

It might be ethically acceptable to consent to family requests, even when not shared by physicians, provided that the choice does not imply risk of harming the patient's dignity or is unacceptable in terms of allocation of resources.

The decision relating to proportionality of treatment is the prerogative of each person, whether they can express their consent/dissent to the treatment or, if incompetent, have prepared ADs. This is even better if in a context of shared care planning (SCP).

The fact that prognostic uncertainty can be reduced but not eliminated should not lead to prognostic paralysis (an alibi for not making decisions) [56].

In this sense, there is no schematic approach applicable to different clinical situations. The possibility of a *"time- or event- or skill-limited"* approach must always be considered.

The decision-making process that leads to treatment limitation must always be clearly and explicitly documented in the medical records [57].

6.7.3 Decision to Forgo Life-Sustaining Treatments: The Goals

The limitation of treatments has the sole purpose of avoiding the prolonging agony, allowing the patient to die from the consequences of their disease. This clearly differs from euthanasia where shortening of the dying process is the intention.

It is clinically appropriate and ethically responsible not to prolong the dying process when approaching the terminal stages of the disease. The treatment-limiting process must minimize the dying patient's suffering and adopt the most suitable approach for the specific clinical situation [45, 46].

DFLST should be considered when:

1. The clinical situation renders treatment continuation inappropriate
2. The patient withdraws or denies their consent
3. There is no response to treatment

The limitation of treatments always implies therapy reassessment towards increased palliative care.

Clinicians have a moral duty to ensure adequate symptom management at the end of life. This can be done through the administration of sedative and analgesic drugs in doses that, theoretically, could shorten the dying person's life [58].

The *double-effect* doctrine morally distinguishes between the administration of drugs aimed at shortening the life of a dying person and the administration of those same drugs to ensure an adequate control of pain and other symptoms (dyspnea, agitation, delirium, nausea), even when high doses are needed [59]. In this case, there is a conscious risk of shortening life even though this is not the purpose.

Some studies have shown that the administration of sedative and analgesic drugs at the end of life does not accelerate the dying process [60].

The aim of deep sedation when administered in the final stages of life should be clearly explained to family members and documented on medical records. According to the clinical response of the dying patient, symptoms and drug dose titrations should be reassessed.

A suitable sedation and analgesic plan must always be formulated, particularly before WDLST, to anticipate the development of intense symptoms [60].

6.7.4 Withdrawing Life-Sustaining Treatments: Basics in Clinical Practice

The abrupt withdrawal of all life-sustaining treatments, except for mechanical ventilation and mechanical circulatory supports, does not induce distress to the patient [46].

Hence, there is no rationale in proceeding to a slow treatment de-escalation, including antibiotics and blood product infusion, hydration, nutrition, and renal replacement therapies.

The timing of suspension for each treatment should be patient-tailored and, in any case, it should be sequential. This can be done by observing the patient's response following the suspension of each treatment, before suspending the next one.

It is recommended to suspend life-sustaining treatments in the following order:

1. Renal replacement therapies
2. Antibiotics, blood products, hydration, and nutrition
3. Vasopressors and/or inotropes, cardiac implantable electronic devices (see Chap. 7 for details), or mechanical circulatory supports (intra-aortic balloon pump, extracorporeal membrane oxygenation, ventricular assist device)
4. Mechanical ventilation

During treatment withdrawing, supplementary oxygen should be administered only if necessary to comfort the dying person [57].

All diagnostic procedures and laboratory tests should be suspended as they are inappropriate and annoying for the patient.

Continuous monitoring must be noninvasive (heart rate, noninvasive blood pressure measurement) to provide patient suffering control and eventual reassessment of sedative and analgesic administration.

Each measurement should be carried out ensuring the dying person's privacy at the bedside. If a long period of suffering is expected in ICU, transfer to a private room should be considered, ICU accommodation availability permitting.

It is mandatory to guarantee deep continuous sedation to the dying patient candidate for WDLST, to prevent or treat symptoms causing suffering (pain, agitation, delirium, respiratory distress) [57].

Doses of sedative and analgesic drugs must be titrated according to the patient's response. The dosage limits coincide with those necessary to obtain suitable symptom control for the whole duration of the EoL stages [57].

A combination of opioids and hypnotics can be used for palliative sedation during the withdrawing of life-sustaining treatments. As with opioids, a bolus dose followed by intravenous infusion is recommended [58].

Withdrawal of mechanical ventilation takes place through progressive reduction of ventilator support until spontaneous respiration is reached [57].

There is a theoretical rationale to gradual weaning from these supports, because rapid reduction of oxygen supply until withdrawal may lead to respiratory distress.

It can be suggested to withdraw mechanical ventilation so as to ensure patient comfort at each step. This may be obtained through gradual reduction of inspired oxygen concentration, ventilator rate, positive end-expiratory pressure, and pressure support [57].

The use of noninvasive ventilation (NIV) in EoL care must be carefully assessed [61]. NIV should be reserved only to cases where drugs did not reach the optimal deep sedation effect (the desired effect) and it should not be routinely used following withdrawal of mechanical ventilation after extubation [52].

## 6.8	Conclusions

The clinical and assistance path for EoL patients is now part of intensive medicine and requires the same levels of knowledge, skill, and experience as all the other areas of activity carried out in the ICU.

The decision to limit the life-sustaining treatments (WHLST or WDLST) is an integral part of this pathway.

As physicians working in an era of great technological and pharmacological advancement, it should be a privilege for us to assist our patients, also during the dying process. Physicians must prevent death from becoming a technological or impersonal event, guaranteeing that those for whom we can do nothing more die in dignity.

This means that there is the need to reassess treatments towards palliation: stopping treatment does not mean stopping care. It means recognizing that for each patient, as with medicine, there is a limit to treatment in terms of rationality (knowledge cannot satisfy all requests), clinical efficacy (a limit that changes with scientific knowledge advancement), and sense (the acceptability of moral choices).

References

1. Rhodes A, Ferdinande P, Flaatten H, Guidet B, Metnitz PG, Moreno RP. The variability of critical care bed numbers in Europe. Intensive Care Med. 2012;38:1647–53.
2. Vincent JL, Marshall JC, Namendys-Silva SA, François B, Martin-Loeches I, Lipman J, et al.; ICON Investigators: Assessment of the worldwide burden of critical illness: the intensive care over nations (ICON) audit. Lancet Respir Med 2014; 2:380–386.
3. Sinha SS, Sjoding MW, Sukul D, Prescott HC, Iwashyna TJ, Gurm HS, et al. Changes in primary non-cardiac diagnoses over time among elderly cardiac intensive care unit patients in the United States. Circ Cardiovasc Qual Outcomes. 2017;10(8):e003616. https://doi.org/10.1161/CIRCOUTCOMES.117.003616.
4. Bonnefoy-Cudraz E, Bueno H, Casella G, De Maria E, Fitzsimons D, Halvorsen S, et al. Acute cardiovascular care association position paper on intensive cardiovascular care units: an update on their definition, structure, organisation and function. Eur Heart J Acute Cardiovasc Care. 2018;7:80–95.
5. Courtney E, Bennett CE, Scott Wright R, Jentzer J, Gajic O, Murphree DH, Murphy JG, et al. Severity of illness assessment with application of the APACHE IV predicted mortality and outcome trends analysis in an academic cardiac intensive care unit. J Crit Care. 2019;50:242–6.
6. Jentzer JC, van Diepen S, Barsness JW, Katz JN, Wiley BM, Bennett CE, et al. Changes in comorbidities, diagnoses, therapies and outcomes in a contemporary cardiac intensive care unit population. Am Heart J. 2019;215:12–9.
7. Berg DD, Bohula EA, van Diepen S, Katz JN, Alviar CL, Baird-Zars VM, et al. Epidemiology of shock in contemporary cardiac intensive care units. Data from the Critical Care Cardiology Trials Network Registry. Circ Cardiovasc Qual Outcomes. 2019;12:e005618. https://doi.org/10.1161/CIRCOUTCOMES.119.005618.
8. Azoulay E, Metnitz B, Sprung CL, Timsit JF, Lemaire F, Bauer P, et al. End-of-life practices in 282 intensive care units: data from the SAPS 3 database. Intensive Care Med. 2009;35:623–30.
9. Sprung CL, Ricou B, Hartog CS, Maia P, Mentzelopoulos SD, Weiss M, et al. Changes in end-of-life practices in European Intensive Care Units from 1999 to 2016. JAMA. 2019;322:1–12.
10. Lobo SM, De Simoni FHB, Jakob SM, Estella A, Vadi S, Bluethgen A, et al.; ICON Investigators. Decision-making on withholding or withdrawing life support in the ICU: a worldwide perspective Chest 2017;152:321–329.
11. Sprung CL, Carmel S, Sjokvist P, Baras M, Cohen SL, Maia P, et al. Attitudes of European physicians, nurses, patients, and families regarding end-of-life decisions: the ETHICATT study. Intensive Care Med. 2007;33:104–10.
12. Curtis JR, Vincent JL. Ethics and end-of-life care for adults in the intensive care unit. Lancet. 2010;376:1347–53.
13. Ay E, Weigand MA, Röhrig R, Gruss M. Dying in the Intensive Care Unit (ICU): a retrospective descriptive analysis of deaths in the ICU in a communal tertiary hospital in Germany. Anesthesiol Res Pract. 2020;2020:2356019. https://doi.org/10.1155/2020/2356019.
14. Sprung CL, Truog RD, Curtis JR, Joynt GM, Baras M, Michalsen A, et al. Seeking worldwide professional consensus on the principles of end-of-life care for the critically ill. The consensus for worldwide end-of-life practice for patients in intensive care units (WELPICUS) study. Am J Respir Crit Care Med. 2014;190:855–66.
15. Vincent JL. Withdrawing may be preferable to witholding. Crit Care. 2005;9:226–9.
16. Garland A, Connors AF. Physicians' influence over decisions to forego life support. J Palliat Med. 2007;10:1298–305.

17. Bülow HH, Sprung CL, Baras M, Carmel S, Svantesson M, Benbenishty J, et al. Are reli-gion and religiosity important to end-of-life decisions and patient autonomy in the ICU? The Ethicatt study. Intensive Care Med. 2012;38:1126–33.
18. Eidelman LA, Jakobson DJ, Pizov R, Geber D, Leibovitz L, Sprung CL. Forgoing life-sustaining treatment in an Israeli UTI. Intensive Care Med. 1998;24:162–6.
19. Aldawood AS, Alsultan M, Arabi YM, Baharoon SA, Al-Qahtani S, Haddad SH, et al. End-of-life practices in a tertiary intensive care unit in Saudi Arabia. Anaesth Intensive Care. 2012;40:137–41.
20. Yazigi A, Riachi M, Dabbar G. Withholding and withdrawal of life-sustaining treatment in a Lebanese intensive care unit: a prospective observational study. Intensive Care Med. 2005;31:562–7.
21. Mani RK, Mandal AK, Bal S, Javeri Y, Kumar R, Nama DK, et al. End-of-life decisions in an Indian intensive care unit. Intensive Care Med. 2009;35:1713–9.
22. McLean RF, Tarshis J, Mazer CD, Szalai JP. Death in two Canadian intensive care units: insti-tutional difference and changes over time. Crit Care Med. 2000;28:100–3.
23. White DB, Curtis JR, Lo B, Luce JM. Decisions to limit life-sustaining treatment for critically ill patients who lack both decision-making capacity and surrogate decision-makers. Crit Care Med. 2006;34:2053–9.
24. Cooper Z, Rivara FP, Wang J, Mackenzie EJ, Jurkovich GJ. Withdrawal of life-sustaining ther-apy in injured patients: variations between trauma centers and nontrauma centers. J Trauma. 2009;66:1327–35.
25. Ferrand E, Robert R, Ingrand P, Lemaire F. Withholding and withdrawal of life support in intensive care units in France: a prospective survey. French LATAREA Group. Lancet. 2001;357:9–14.
26. Wunsch H, Harrison DA, Harvey S, Rowan K. End-of-life decisions: a cohort study of the withdrawal of all active treatment in intensive care units in the United Kingdom. Intensive Care Med. 2005;31:823–31.
27. Prendergast TJ, Claessens MT, Luce JM. A national survey of end-of-life care for critically ill patients. Am J Respir Crit Care Med. 1998;158:1163–7.
28. Quill CM, Ratcliffe SJ, Harhay MO, Halpern SD. Variation in decisions to forgo life-sustaining therapies in US ICU. Chest. 2014;146:573–82.
29. Giannini A, Pessina A, Tacchi EM. End-of-life decisions in intensive care units: attitudes of physicians in an Italian urban setting. Intensive Care Med. 2003;29:1902–10.
30. Bertolini G, Boffelli S, Malacarne P, Peta M, Marchesi M, Barbisan C, et al. End-of-life decision-making and quality of ICU performance: an observational study in 84 Italian units. Intensive Care Med. 2010;36:1495–504.
31. Giacomini M, Cook D, DeJean D, Shaw R, Gedge E. Decision tools for life support: a review and policy analysis. Crit Care Med. 2006;34:864–70.
32. Sprung CL, Paruk F, Sa F, Hartog CS, Lipman J, Du B, et al. The Durban World Congress Ethics Round Table Conference Report: differences between withholding and withdrawing life-sustaining treatments. J Crit Care. 2014;29:890–5.
33. Sulmasy DP, Sugarman J. Are withholding and withdrawing therapy always morally equiva-lent? J Med Ethics. 1994;20:218–22.
34. Bostrom N, Ord T. The reversal test: eliminating status quo bias in applied ethics. Ethics. 2006;116:656–79.
35. Doing vs allowing harm. The Stanford encyclopedia of philosophy; 2016. http://stanford.io/2kSkzRw. Accessed Feb 2020.
36. Christakis NA, Asch DA. Biases in how physicians choose to withdraw life support. Lancet. 1993;342:642–6.
37. Persad G, Wertheimer A, Emanuel EJ. Principles for allocation of scarce medical interven-tions. Lancet. 2009;373:423–31.
38. American Thoracic Society. Fair allocation of intensive care unit resources. Am J Respir Crit Care Med. 1997;156:1282–301.

39. Riccioni L, Busca MT, Busatta L, Orsi L, Gristina GR. Forgoing treatments: a kind of euthanasia? A scientific approach to the debate about end of life decisions. Recenti Prog Med. 2016;107:127–39.

40. Smedira NG, Evans BH, Grais LS, Cohen NH, Lo B, Cooke M, et al. Withholding and withdrawal of life support from the critically ill. N Engl J Med. 1990;322:309–15.

41. Simchen E, Sprung CL, Galai N, Zitser-Gurevich Y, Bar-Lavi Y, Levi L, et al. Survival of critically ill patients hospitalized in and out of intensive care. Crit Care Med. 2007;35:449–57.

42. Biston P, Aldecoa C, Devriendt J, Madl C, Chochrad D, Vincent JL, et al. Outcome of elderly patients with circulatory failure. Intensive Care Med. 2014;40:50–6.

43. Guidet B, Flaatten H, Boumendil A, Morandi A, Andersen FH, Artigas A, et al.; VIP1 Study Group. Withholding or withdrawing of life-sustaining therapy in older adults (≥80 years) admitted to the intensive care unit. Intensive Care Med. 2018;44:1027–1038.

44. Zaal IJ, Devlin JW, Peelen LM, Slooter AJC. A systematic review of risk factors for delirium in the ICU. Crit Care Med. 2015;43:40–7.

45. Iwashyna TJ, Ely EW, Smith DM, Langa KM. Long-term cognitive impairment and functional disability among survivors of severe sepsis. JAMA. 2010;304:1787–94.

46. Bagshaw SM, Stelfox HT, McDermid RC, Rolfson DB, Tsuyuki RT, Baig N, et al. Association between frailty and short- and long-term outcomes among critically ill patients: a multicentre prospective cohort study. CMAJ. 2014;186:E95–102.

47. Jackson JC, Pandharipande PP, Girard TD, Brummel NE, Thompson JL, Hughes CG, et al. Depression, post-traumatic stress disorder, and functional disability in survivors of critical illness in the BRAIN-ICU study: a longitudinal cohort study. Lancet Respir Med. 2014;2:369–79.

48. Kahn JM, Angus DC, Cox CE, Hough CL, White DB, Yende S, et al. The epidemiology of chronic critical illness in the United States. Crit Care Med. 2015;43:282–7.

49. Douglas SL, Daly BJ, Lipson AR. Neglect of quality-of-life considerations in intensive care unit family meetings for long-stay intensive care unit patients. Crit Care Med. 2012;40:461–7.

50. Sprung CL, Danis M, Iapichino G, Artigas A, Kesecioglu J, Moreno R, et al. Triage of intensive care patients: identifying agreement and controversy. Intensive Care Med. 2013;39:1916–24.

51. Garrouste-Orgeas M, Tabah A, Vesin A, Philippart F, Kpodji A, Bruel C, et al. The ETHICA study (part II): simulation study of determinants and variability of ICU physician decisions in patients aged 80 or over. Intensive Care Med. 2013;39:1574–83.

52. Marchioni A, Fantini R, Antenora F, Clini E, Fabbri L. Chronic critical illness: the price of survival. Eur J Clin Investig. 2015;45:1341–9.

53. Kentish-Barnes N, Seegers V, Legriel S, Cariou JS, Lefrant JY, et al. CAESAR: a new tool to assess relatives' experience of dying and death in the ICU. Intensive Care Med. 2016;42:995–1002.

54. Kon AA, Shepard EK, Sederstrom NO, Swoboda SM, Marshall MF, Birriel B, et al. Defining futile and potentially inappropriate interventions: a policy statement from the Society of Critical Care Medicine Ethics Committee. Crit Care Med. 2016;44:1769–74.

55. SIAARTI (Società Italiana Anestesia Analgesia Rianimazione Terapia Intensiva). Recommendations for the approach to dying person; Update 2018. https://bit.ly/34GmhvI. Accessed Feb 2020.

56. Smith AK, White DB, Arnold RM. Uncertainty—the other side of prognosis. N Engl J Med. 2013;368:2448–50.

57. Bosslet GT, Pope TM, Rubenfeld GD, Lo B, Truog RD, Rushton CH, et al. An official ATS/AACN/ACCP/ESICM/SCCM policy statement: responding to requests for potentially inappropriate treatments in intensive care units. Am J Respir Crit Care Med. 2015;191:1318–30.

58. Downar J, Delaney JW, Hawryluck L, Kenny L. Guidelines for the withdrawal of life-sustaining measures. Intensive Care Med. 2016;42:1003–17.

59. Truog RD, Campbell ML, Curtis JR, Haas CE, Luce JM, Rubenfeld GD, et al. Recommendations for end-of-life care in the intensive care unit: a consensus statement by the American College of Critical Care Medicine. Crit Care Med. 2008;36:953–63.

60. Canadian Critical Care Society Ethics Committee, Bandrauk N, Downar J, Paunovic B. Withholding and withdrawing life-sustaining treatment: The Canadian Critical Care Society position paper. Can J Anaesth. 2018;65:105–22.
61. Curtis JR, Cook DJ, Sinuff T, Douglas B, White DB, Hill N, et al. Society of Critical Care Medicine Palliative Non-invasive Positive Ventilation Task Force. Non-invasive positive pressure ventilation in critical and palliative care settings: understanding the goals of therapy. Crit Care Med. 2007;35:932–9.

Deactivation of Cardiac Implantable Electronic Devices (CIEDs) at the End of Life

7

Massimo Romanò

7.1 Introduction

Patients with left ventricular dysfunction may benefit from pharmacological, interventional and surgical treatments, and from dedicated cardiac implantable electronic devices (CIEDs).

These devices include Implantable Cardioverter Defibrillators (ICDs) to prevent sudden cardiac death, Cardiac Resynchronisation Therapy (CRT) in patients with complete left bundle branch block (LBBB), eventually associated with ICD (CRT-D), and normal pacemakers (PM) to treat bradyarrhythmias [1].

When the patient's condition worsens, at the final stages of life (multiple-organ failure, acute cerebrovascular events, cancer, chronic neurological diseases, etc.) the question may arise whether to deactivate these devices or to leave them active until the patient's death [2–6].

This is especially true for patients with ICDs as they might receive frequent and painful shocks from the device, in the last stages of life.

The deactivation choice comes along with different clinical, ethical and relational issues specific to the different devices.

Cardiologists are generally late in dealing with these issues due to their cultural, training and emotional reasons [7, 8]. They feel great discomfort initiating discussion on treatment choices with patients and family members at the end of life (EoL) [9].

This compromises optimal patient care due to the inadequate attention to the quality of life and needs of advanced/terminally ill patients, particularly those with HF.

M. Romanò (✉)
Organizing Committee, Postgraduate Master In Palliative Care, University of Milan, Milano, Italy
e-mail: max.romano51@gmail.com

When dealing with CIED deactivation, clinicians must comply with medical ethics principles, with special attention on the principle of patient autonomy [10].

7.2 Implantable Cardioverter-Defibrillators (ICDs)

ICD implants for primary prevention of sudden cardiac death are advised for patients with post-infarction left ventricular dysfunction or patients affected by HF of any aetiology [11, 12], even with more recent reassessment in patients with non-ischaemic HF [13].

The incidence of HF patients' sudden death has significantly reduced thanks to pharmacological, ICD and CRT therapies. However, the correct selection of patients to be submitted to ICD implants is an increasingly more relevant problem [14, 15].

The most recent available data reports about 737,000 new ICD implants and over 254,000 ICD replacements worldwide each year [16, 17].

Total ICD implants in Italy in 2018 amount to 18,353 (13,994 first implants and 4359 replacements) [18].

In the Madit II study [19] the relative risk of death at 20 months in patients with post-infarction left ventricular dysfunction and with ICD implants is reduced by 31%, compared to a conventional treatment group, the absolute risk is reduced by 5.6%, while at 8 years the relative risk is reduced by 34% and the absolute risk by 13% [20].

In patients with heart failure, the relative risk of death is reduced by 23% and the absolute risk by 7.2% at 5 years [21].

The annual percentage of delivered shocks (appropriate and inappropriate) varies according to the main studies: it registers 7.5% in the SCD-HeFT study [21] (randomised trial, with a mean follow-up of 5 years), with an annual 5.1% of appropriate shock on malignant ventricular tachyarrhythmias, while in a wide-ranging Swedish study [22] (3-year mean follow-up) the total yearly shock percentage was 8.4% (appropriate shock 6%/year, inappropriate shock 2.4%/year).

During a long-term follow-up patients implanted with ICDs as primary prevention will in most cases experience a non-arrhythmic death due to the progression of the heart disease or other severe pathologies, for instance organ failure, cancer, degenerative neurological diseases and dementia, without the device ever delivering appropriate shocks until the last weeks or days of life.

In a study that analysed ICD memory data in 125 deceased patients suffering from HF, death due to arrhythmias occurred in a minority of cases (13%), while 37% of deaths were secondary to the progression of HF and 38% to non-cardiac causes [23].

The prolonging of arrhythmia detection time allows a reduction in the total number of shocks, appropriate and inappropriate, and a greater use of antitachycardia therapy [24].

However, implants are linked to anxiety and depression in about 20% of patients [25]. This percentage doubles in patients that have received shocks, appropriate and inappropriate, with a dose-response relationship: the more shocks received, the

Table 7.1 Incidence of ICD shock at the end of life

Author	Source	Patients	% of shock	Time lapse
Goldstein [27]	Relatives	100	20%	Weeks/days/hours
Goldstein [28]	Hospice	nd	58%	Last year
Sherazi [29]	Madit II	98	15%	Last weeks
Kinch-Westerdhal [23]	ICD	125	31%	Last hours (arrhythmic storm 24%)
Trussler [55]	ICD	50	20%	Last month

greater the anxiety. The intense pain caused by the shock, a sense of insecurity and more generally a fear of death are the main causes for this psychological reaction [26].

The main issue is whether and how to proceed with ICD deactivation in patients with severe deterioration of their general clinical conditions and at the EoL. In fact, patients are at risk of receiving painful and frequent shocks with no significant survival advantage, but with a worsening of their quality of life.

To solve the issue, ICD shock frequency in the last stages of life needs first to be analysed: Table 7.1 shows data from the main surveys dealing with EoL shock frequency. It emerges that shocks are far more frequent in the last days or hours of life, often with the characteristics of an arrhythmic storm.

The problems with ICD deactivation in EoL patients, supported by Scientific Societies recommendations [2, 3, 9], are more than present [23, 27–33].

7.2.1 Ethical Problems

One of the queries relating to EoL ICD deactivation refers to the nature of a cardiac device once it has been implanted.

Is the device an indivisible part of the patient? If so, does the deactivation result in a euthanasia-type action?

On this matter Scientific Societies recommendations [2, 3] take up and state Daniel Sulmasy's thesis [34, 35] where distinctions are made between the different forms of treatment.

According to Sulmasy, 'all therapies intending to restore health can be classified in two different ways: regulative and constitutive'. 'Regulative' treatment aims at returning the organism to its own homeostatic equilibrium. This is the case, for example, for antiarrhythmic or antipyretic drugs, and ICD. The 'constitutive' treatment takes over the function that the body can no longer carry out by itself (see Fig. 7.1).

'Constitutive' therapies can further be distinguished into replacement or substitutive therapies: replacement therapy is a treatment that becomes an integral part of the body and completely replaces a lost physiological function (organ transplant, artificial heart valve). Substitutive therapy, on the other hand, refers to a function substitution, in a different manner to what occurs in a healthy person (dialysis,

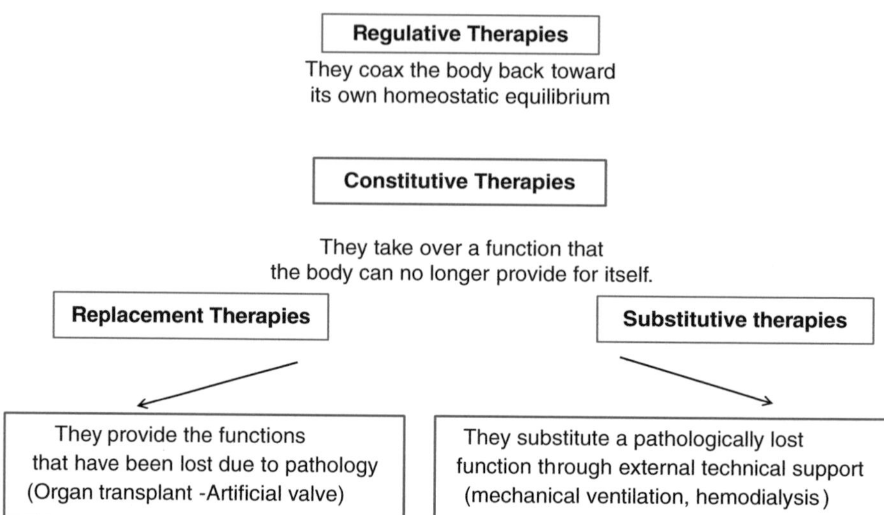

Fig. 7.1 Different definitions of treatment and their bioethics meaning. Sulmasy D. [34] modified

mechanical ventilation, mechanical circulatory support); it does not become a part of the patient and needs external technical support.

These distinctions can support the decision to deactivate a device or not [34–36]. It is unethical to 'deactivate' an organ transplant, for example by administering drugs that are potentially lethal for the organ, whereas it is ethical with dialysis or mechanical ventilation, in specific clinical contexts, especially at the end of life [37].

ICDs are generally identified as regulative [2, 3, 23, 27, 30, 31, 33] as they return the abnormal cardiac rhythm to normal sinus rhythm. Based on this regulative action, their deactivation may be considered ethical.

EoL ICD deactivation can be supported by various ethical reasons, from both principlism and sanctity/inviolability of life ethics.

The first refers to four bioethics principles: autonomy and self-determination (respect the patient's decisions), beneficence (propose good for the patient), non-maleficence (*primum non nocere*—do no harm) and distributive justice (guarantee the patient's free access to available treatments and the equal distribution of economic and human resources available). ICD deactivation is morally acceptable if it respects patient autonomy and promotes good for the patient avoiding any harm [38].

The second, sanctity of life ethics, is characterised by the prohibition of interference with the finalism intrinsic to human life [39].

In this ethical vision the justification for ICD deactivation is based on the double-effect doctrine. It is morally lawful to carry out a treatment that has a positive effect (alleviating suffering) and a possible negative effect (hypothetical shortening of life), provided that certain requirements are respected:

1. The causative action is not in itself bad, but good or neutral.
2. The good and bad effects both take place contemporarily to the action, i.e. the good effect is not obtained by or from the bad effect.

3. The intention is oriented towards good or good effect; the bad effect is not sought but is only expected or permitted.
4. The relationship between the desired good effect and the bad tolerated effect is reasonably proportionate.

Contrary opinion to ICD deactivation does not seem to emerge from the various religious orientations [40].

At the ethical level, the deactivation of an ICD is thus a possible option and coherent with the EoL palliative approach. Death is not immediate; it is due to the final progression of the underlying disease, not due to the introduction of a new pathology or the intention to actively induce the end of the patient's life, even if in agreement with the patient. Thus, it is completely different from euthanasia or assisted suicide [34, 35].

In general, physicians and bioethicists agree on different meanings of 'killing' and 'allowing to die', even if with some differences.

Karches and Sulmasy define it as: 'An act of killing creates a new, lethal, patho-logic state in a human being with the intention of causing death, whereas an act of allowing to die occurs when a physician withholds or withdraws a treatment of a preexisting fatal disease, foreseeing the patient's likely death. Acts of allowing to die can sometimes be morally justified. The intention must be to end the treatment, not the patient' [36].

All the authors highlight the importance of sharing the decision with the patients and respecting their autonomy, regardless of the meanings attributed to the device. Accordingly this should be the only element to consider for an ethical judgment [2, 3, 10, 30, 31]. Autonomy of the competent patient is the overriding principle in any decision.

In incompetent patients, the choice relating to ICD deactivation should follow a hierarchical scale consisting of [41]:

1. Advance directives.
2. In the absence of advance directives, the so-called substituted judgement (that is, the desires and wishes previously expressed by the patient to family members or the care team) must be adopted, while taking into account the practical difficul-ties that this situation sometimes entails [41].
3. In the absence of the two preceding conditions, the patient's best interest is iden-tified, based on the balance between expected benefits and treatment burden, according to the principle of proportionality.

It is clearly unethical to unilaterally decide to deactivate an ICD against the will of the patient, family members or surrogate decision maker, even when the doctor considers it futile maintaining it active [42, 43].

A related issue is whether or not to replace an ICD due to end of battery life, particularly in the elderly. Here it is considered correct to generally reassess the case due to possible variations in the clinical picture that led to the first implant and to balance the relationship between treatment aims, quality of life, costs and risk of complications from ICD replacement [44].

Moreover, in patients undergoing generator replacement, the residual risk of appropriate shocks is not negligible, even in elderly patients, in the absence of intervention during the first implant [45]; this can occur even with only moderate left ventricular dysfunction [46].

7.2.2 Information and Patient Awareness

There is a broad gap between what patients should know and what they actually know about the final stages of life, and hence what they need to know about ICD management [47]. This is reflected in a broad and heterogenous range of patient and physician behaviour.

In a wide-ranging Swedish register of over 2400 patients with ICDs, 40% of patients did not want to discuss either their disease trajectory or device deactivation, regardless of the presence of HF [47]. The willingness to discuss increases only in cases of repeated shocks, high levels of anxiety or concern related to the presence of ICD. Similarly, also the clinician's willingness is limited.

Patient perplexities or opposition [48] to device deactivation is generally due to a lack of information on the real impact of the ICD on the quality and duration of life, and due to differing opinions on EoL deactivation.

Patients generally overestimate HF prognosis compared to risk scores, even in the more advanced stages of the disease [49].

In many cases, the obstacles to shared care planning (SCP) in patients with CIEDs are secondary to a combination of factors. These include the overestimation of the impact that the devices themselves can have on disease progression and probability of dying, the lack of patient-doctor communication and the relationship with technological progress presupposing the infallibility of devices in preventing death, defined by some as the *biotechnical embrace* [50]. In short, information is generally incomplete and scant.

This data confirms what emerges from the study by Stewart et al. [51]. It is based on interview reports from 105 enrolled patients according to the SCDHeFT study indications: 65% patients had an ICD for primary prevention of sudden death, of which 82% never received a shock.

Patients were questioned on the quantity of lives they thought ICDs could save over 5 years (in the SCDHeFT study 7.2%): 77% thought it was more than 10 and 54% thought it could be over 50.

When facing hypothetical scenarios in which deactivation could be considered, 70% of patients with ICDs were unwilling, even at the final stages of cancer, 55% also with repeated and daily shocks, and no one was willing to deactivate ICDs also in case of intense suffering from continuous dyspnoea at rest.

ICD deactivation is not even considered among the listed choices in the advance directives (ADs): in the Kinch Westerdhal et al. [23] study, 52% of interviewed patients had expressed ADs, above all the 'do-not-resuscitate' (DNR) order.

Nevertheless, 51% of patients that had given DNR orders still had the ICD active up to 1 h prior to death and the deactivation occurred only in 49% of cases, on average 4 days before death.

In several studies [33, 52–56] in which AD percentages ranged from 30% to 50%, only a minimum percentage of patients (1–8%) had formulated specific ADs allowing ICD deactivation (see Table 7.2), except in one numerically small study where ICD deactivation was included in the AD in 32% of cases [56].

Moreover, (Table 7.2) variable percentages of patients (from 17% to 28%) judged EoL ICD deactivation procedure similar to assisted suicide or to euthanasia [32, 52–56].

The percentage of patients informed of eventual ICD deactivation at the time of implantation is low and a significant number of them would prefer to discuss it at the end of life; however, half of the patients were willing to discuss it at the moment of the implantation (see Table 7.3) [57–59].

What sometimes impacts willingness to discuss and eventually start device deactivation can be the stage of disease or the non-eligibility to advanced treatments, for instance heart transplant or mechanical circulatory support. Effective professional training is needed to improve physicians' communication and thus encourage conversations on deactivation, but still, this does not increase the number of deactivated devices [60].

Table 7.2 Patient opinions and preferences on end-of-life ICD deactivation

Author	Patients	Assisted suicide/ Euthanasia	Advance Directives	Advance Directives/ ICD
Kirkpatrick [33]	278	26%	51%	2%
Tajouri [52]	420	nd	30%	2%
Stromberg [53]	3067	28%	nd	nd
Kramer [54]	546	17%	47%	8%
Buchalter [55]	150	nd	57%	0.75%
Trussler [56]	49	nd	41%	32%

Table 7.3 Patient opinions and preferences on end-of-life ICD deactivation information

Author	Patients	Informed at moment of implantation?	Discussed at moment of implantation?	Discussed at end of life?
Raphael [57]	54	38%	40%	21%
Thylen [58]	3067	14%	50%	69%
Pedersen [59]	294	28%	49%	26%

A separate case is that of the very elderly (octogenarians or nonagenarians), a quarter of whom do not have sufficient information on ICD functioning, nor on the ethical and practical aspects of deactivation. Only 13% had discussed it with their doctor or family members. The majority desired a replacement even if they were old or gravely ill and 30% wished the ICD to be active, despite the chance of receiving a shock in the final stages of disease [61].

Around one-third of patients had discussed the possible disease trajectory with their doctor; this significantly increased the willingness to deactivation. Thanks to discussions on ICD deactivation, the last decade has witnessed a rise in willingness to discuss it (from 6% to 35%), as with the actual number of deactivations (from 16% to 42%); nevertheless, the majority of patients die with active devices [56, 62].

On the other hand, there are reports where the majority of interviewees state to be interested not only in discussion, but also in approving the decision to deactivate the ICD at the end of life [57, 59, 63].

In this complex, variable and evolving situation, with a large number of patients unwilling to discuss the disease trajectory and EoL decisions (including the deactivation of a life-saving device), how should we position ourselves?

We should respect the patient's choices without prevarication, improving our communication skills with the goal of increasing patient awareness, achieving transparent shared decision-making ensuring patient-informed choices [56, 60].

7.2.3 The Opinion of Physicians and Nurses

There is a great deal of evidence that physicians do not fully have the communication tools to properly address these issues with the patient and family members [7] and perceive even the possibility of deactivating an implanted device as negative [64].

The Scientific Societies documents [2, 3] suggest that the decision to deactivate an ICD must be the result of a shared process between the physician, the patient and the family members. It should become part of a discussion on the possible illness trajectory. Finally it should be integrated within a shared decision-making process and initiated early (preferably at the time of the implantation) and not at the end of life.

However, this happens rarely and irregularly [65], as reported by the different surveys carried out, with misperceptions of ethical and legal aspects.

The distress experienced by physicians during ICD deactivation talks is intense, more than that dealing with the withdrawal of other life support treatments, namely dialysis or mechanical ventilation. 48% consider ICD deactivation as ethically different to those procedures and 20% believe that the decision might have legal consequences [7].

However, at least in intention, many physicians (56–83%) would start discussing ICD deactivation in cases of terminal illness, which is still less than those willing to discuss advance directives or DNR (82–94%) [66].

In other surveys, 10–20% of doctors considered deactivation unethical, analogous to assisted suicide or euthanasia, and over 40% judged it illegal [67, 68].

In a survey carried out in 47 European centres [69], 85% of cardiologists reported to have discussed deactivation only in specific cases, whereas 62% thought it correct to discuss it with the patient at the end of life.

In a more recent study [70], 79% of the doctors interviewed did not feel uncomfortable thinking of discussing ICD deactivation with the patient and 35% stated doing so routinely.

Most distressed are the younger doctors, with only 16% usually discussing it with the patient. 21% of those interviewed erroneously believed that DNR orders are equivalent to the deactivation request.

Training to improve communication with patients has produced contrasting results.

Choi et al. have reported positive results from 6 months' teaching sessions with cardiologists and two groups of patients, regarding ICD deactivation. The first group had expressed a DNR order and the other would receive palliative care. At the end of the sessions, the percentage of patients that had discussed deactivation increased from 32% to 70% in the DNR group and from 50% to 93% in the palliative care group. In parallel, the percentage of ICD deactivation increased from 29% to 40% in the DNR group and from 45% to 73% in the palliative care group [71].

In another recent study, despite basal high self-assessment rating, based on trust and skill in discussion on ACP, an ad hoc physician training did not produce significant improvement after 3 months [72].

Although palliativists are largely favourable to ICD deactivation, they point out a lack of experience in starting the discussion, together with a lack of familiarity with specific shared protocols [66].

A key but sometimes neglected professional figure in EoL decisions for patients with ICD is the nursing team.

Nurses consider information received by the patients on ADs and ICD deactivation as insufficient. They think, in contrast to what has been accepted up to now in biomedical ethics, that there is a difference between withholding a treatment and withdrawing one, and consider ICD deactivation as being acceptable in EoL patients only after all the other treatments have been withdrawn. In any case, ICD deactivation comes along with suffering [73].

The practice varies from country to country. US physicians and nurses are more inclined to deactivation discussion compared to Europeans. However, nurses are more reluctant and feel less secure compared to doctors [74].

A similar situation (roles and ethical conflicts) is also experienced by industry representatives, when, in the absence of skilled physicians, they are involved in ICD deactivation procedures (more common in North America than in Europe) [75].

A common fact emerges from the surveys reported in literature: ICD deactivation can only occur 'peacefully' if it is within a process discussed over time with the patient. Consideration should start in the pre-implant stage, in an informed way and within a schedule that progressively deals with issues relating to prognosis, allowing complete and shared care planning, including ADs.

In conclusion:

1. Patients with ICD in the final stage of life frequently receive repeated, painful shocks which cannot change the evolution of the underlying illness.
2. Patients are often reluctant, if not contrary, to discussing EoL decisions and issues, generally due to a lack of complete information on the efficacy of cardiac implanted devices and the problems connected to their management. They do not receive adequate information in the pre-implant stage nor during follow-up. They are more willing to deactivation when they have received repeated shocks and have a bad quality of life.
3. Physicians are unprepared in the discussion of these issues; their relationship with the patient could profoundly change by improving communication skills.

The Heart Rhythm Society (HRS) and the European Heart Rhythm Association (EHRA) consensus documents [2, 3] provide some behavioural suggestions:

1. ICD deactivation must be the final point of a transparent and well-deliberated process, with full and documented traceability (also written) of the decisions taken by the patient and the physician.
2. If the conscience clause is invoked by the physician and/or industry representative, another physician or industry representative must be available.
3. The possibility to deactivate an ICD, when the disease worsens, should be discussed with the patient at the moment of implant and be an integral part of informed consent including specific references and sentences concerning the situations in which to proceed with deactivation.
4. The patient that chooses to deactivate an ICD must be guaranteed that eventual reconsideration will be accepted, and the device reactivated.
5. It is possible to deactivate only ICD shock and maintain the antitachycardia therapies that do not determine symptoms, bearing in mind that sometimes they can accelerate the ventricular tachycardia frequency, leading to ventricular fibrillation.
6. In case of arrhythmic storm, if deactivation cannot be arranged, the application of a magnet over the device allows temporary deactivation of shock delivery, leaving the anti-bradycardia pacing unaltered.

7.3   Cardiac Pacemaker (PM)-Cardiac Resynchronisation Therapy-Pacemaker (CRT-P)

PMs can deliver continuous pacing (in PM-dependent patients or in patients with CRT-P) or intermittent pacing (in non-PM-dependent patients).

Queries relating to deactivation in the final stages of life can be posed also with these devices.

PM or CRT-P deactivation has partially different ethical and clinical issues compared to ICDs or CRT-Ds.

First of all, they do not cause symptoms that could interfere with the patient's quality of life.

Secondly, in CRT-P or in non-PM-dependent patients, device deactivation is not to be considered. This is because the clinical picture could be worsened by the symptomatic bradycardia following deactivation, with hemodynamic deterioration, contradicting one basic principle of palliative care, namely to guarantee the best quality of life for the dying person.

The choice of deactivating the PM or CRT-P in PM-dependent patients is ethically controversial, as the deactivation would lead to almost immediate patient death [10, 76, 77].

HRS recommendations [2] do not discriminate between ICDs and PMs on the ethical level, considering that the request to deactivate the devices by the competent patient (or by surrogate decision maker, if the patient is incompetent) is to be satisfied according to the principle of autonomy [31, 36].

EHRA recommendations [3] are more elusive on this issue, due to different sensitivities and legislation in European countries. It must be noted that in Italy the recent 219/2017 law has recognised the individual's faculty to dispose of their own body, their own health and their own life via informed consent (IC), shared care planning and ADs [78].

The number of papers relating to PM deactivation are far more infrequent in literature, compared to those dealing with ICD deactivation. This is probably due to the significant psychological impact involved with PM deactivation. According to the majority of authors, there is no difference between PM deactivation in a PM-dependent patient and withdrawing mechanical ventilation or renal replacement therapies (defined by Sulmasy as substitutive therapies [34]), in specific clinical conditions [7, 36].

The PM-dependent patient's request to deactivate the device must be evaluated not only in respect of his/her decisional autonomy, but also in the context of the patient's burden of suffering, accompanying symptoms and quality of life, which are not influenced by PM [36].

The cause of death may occur from the underlying disease, and not from PM deactivation.

According to other authors, instead, PMs should be referred to as replacement therapies and should not be deactivated, as in this case the patient's death would be caused by an external intervention not related to the underlying disease, leading to a condition similar to euthanasia [10, 77, 78].

7.4   Conclusions

EoL conversations are complex, particularly regarding the management of life support treatments and CIEDs.

As there are no standardised approaches, it would certainly be useful if hospitals define specific protocols, with the aim of establishing with which patients, when and in what ways it is necessary to start the conversation [79].

According to the Scientific Societies recommendations [2, 3], the discussion on the possibility of deactivating a CIED should start before device implantation, be part of IC and continue over time (continuous informed consent), with periodic updates in relation to the evolution of the clinical picture [9].

This creates anxiety in the physician suggesting the implant and confusion in the patient receiving the apparently contradictory message: 'I am proposing the implant of a lifesaving device and at the same time I am talking to you about the possibility of deactivating it in the future' [80].

However, physicians cannot hide the problems deriving from the implanted CIED in specific clinical conditions from patients and their family members.

Discussion on CIED deactivation should also be started at the time of device replacement, if there is life-limiting disease diagnosis or a patient enters a palliative care programme.

The later the discussion begins, the more difficult it will be to explain to the patient the complexity of the decision-making process.

In order to adequately deal with this problem, specific training programmes for all cardiologists should be mandatory. When managing difficult and complex conversations, support from an expert palliative care consultant should be granted.

Finally, there is a crucial element that has not yet been well addressed in literature. Technological evolution offers the patient higher probability to overcome very critical stages of the disease; however, the overestimation of the technological potential has triggered two possible negative and closely linked consequences: the treatment imperative and the technological imperative.

The treatment imperative potentially leads to treatments that are unlikely to bring any clinical benefits.

The technological imperative refers to the physician's attitude to the employment of certain therapies because they are available, even if not recommended, within the logic of doing whatever and everything possible, which can also occur in a self-referential way [81].

This influences the choices and decisions of cardiologists and patients.

The ethical questions at the root of the choices to deactivate a CIED can be analysed based on a moral algorithm centred on specific questions. Even though it was proposed 20 years ago by Edmund Pellegrino, [82] the algorithm is still relevant today [36].

1. **Who decides?** As previously discussed, the decision is primarily taken by the competent patient (the principle of autonomy) and, if not, according to ADs, the presence of a surrogate decision maker or a durable power of attorney. In their absence, substituted judgement is a crucial element [41].
2. **With what criteria?** The basic criterion is related to clinical treatment futility, with all the problems connected to its definition [83]. The main elements are treatment efficacy in relation to the stage of the disease and its natural course; the benefits connected to treatment; the economic burden; the clinical and psychological burden for the patient and their quality of life; and the patient's age.

3. **How to resolve conflicts and prevent them?** Discussion within the healthcare team and with the patient, family members and eventual surrogate decision makers is a fundamental prerequisite to answering positively to queries. Ethical, psychological and religious consultation can be essential elements of support in the most complex cases.

In the absence of the two preceding conditions, the best interest of the patient is identified, based on the balance between expected benefits and treatment severity, according to the principle of proportionality.

References

1. Ponikowski P, Voors AA, Anker SD, et al. 2016 ESC guidelines for the diagnosis and treatment of acute and chronic heart failure: the Task Force for the diagnosis and treatment of acute and chronic heart failure of the European Society of Cardiology. Eur Heart J. 2016;37:2129–200.
2. Lampert R, Hayes DL, Annas GJ, Farley MA, Goldstein NE, Hamilton RM, et al. American College of Cardiology; American Geriatrics Society; American Academy of Hospice and Palliative Medicine; American Heart Association; European Heart Rhythm Association; Hospice and Palliative Nurses Association. HRS Expert Consensus Statement on the management of cardiovascular implantable electronic devices (CIEDs) in patients nearing end of life or requesting withdrawal of therapy. Heart Rhythm. 2010;7:1008–26.
3. Padeletti L, Arnar DO, Boncinelli L, Brachman J, Camm JA, Daubert JC, et al. EHRA Expert Consensus Statement on the management of cardiovascular implantable electronic devices in patients nearing end of life or requesting withdrawal of therapy. Europace. 2010;12:1480–9.
4. Romanò M, Gorni G. Implantable cardiac device deactivation at the end of life. G Ital Cardiol (Rome). 2020;21:286–95.
5. Wordingham SE, McIlvennan CK. Palliative care for patients on mechanical circulatory support. AMA J Ethics. 2019;21:435–42.
6. Klinedinst R, Kornfield ZN, Hadler RA. Palliative care for patients with advanced heart disease. J Cardiothorac Vasc Anesth. 2019;33:833–43.
7. Kramer DB, Kesselheim AS, Brock DW, Maisel WH. Ethical and legal views of physicians regarding deactivation of cardiac implantable electrical devices: a quantitative assessment. Heart Rhythm. 2010;7:1537–42.
8. Sonntag EA, Shah KB, Katz JN. Educating resident and fellow physicians on the ethics of mechanical circulatory support. AMA J Ethics. 2019;21:407–15.
9. Allen L, Stevenson LW, Grady KL, et al. Decision making in advanced heart failure: a scientific statement from the American Heart Association. Circulation. 2012;125:1928–52.
10. Kay GN, Bittner GT. Should implantable cardioverter-defibrillators and permanent pacemakers in patients with terminal illness be deactivated? Circ Arrhythm Electrophysiol. 2009;2:336–9.
11. Priori SG, Blomström-Lundqvist C, Mazzanti A, et al. 2015 ESC Guidelines for the management of patients with ventricular arrhythmias and the prevention of sudden cardiac death: The Task Force for the Management of patients with ventricular arrhythmias and the prevention of sudden cardiac death of the European Society of Cardiology (ESC). Eur Heart J. 2015;36:2793–867.
12. Al-Khatib SM, Stevenson WG, Ackerman MJ, et al. 2017 AHA/ACC/HRS Guideline for management of patients with ventricular arrhythmias and the prevention of sudden cardiac death: a report of the American College of Cardiology/American Heart Association Task Force on Clinical Practice Guidelines and the Heart Rhythm Society. J Am Coll Cardiol. 2018;72:e91–e220.

13. Køber L, Thune JJ, Nielsen JC, Haarbo J, et al. DANISH Investigators. Defibrillator implantation in patients with nonischemic systolic heart failure. N Engl J Med. 2016;375:1221–30.
14. Shen L, Jhund PS, Petrie MC, Claggett BL, Barlera S, Cleland JG, et al. Declining risk of sudden death in heart failure. N Engl J Med. 2017;377:41–51.
15. Packer M. Major reduction in the risk of sudden cardiac death in patients with chronic heart failure with the use of drug and device combinations that favourably affect left ventricular structure. Eur J Heart Fail. 2019;21:823–6.
16. Kremers MS, Hammill SC, Berul CI, et al. The national ICD registry report: version 2.1 including leads and pediatrics for years 2010 and 2011. Heart Rhythm. 2013;10:e59–65.
17. Mond HG, Proclemer A. The 11th world survey of cardiac pacing and implantable cardioverter-defibrillators: calendar year 2009—a World Society of Arrhythmia's project. Pacing Clin Electrophysiol. 2011;34:1013–27.
18. Proclemer A, Zecchin M, D'Onofrio A, Boriani G, Ricci RP, Rebellato L, et al. The Pacemaker and Implantable Cardioverter-Defibrillator Registry of the Italian Association of Arrhythmology and Cardiac Pacing—annual report 2018. G Ital Cardiol. 2020;21:157–69.
19. Moss AJ, Zareba W, Hall WJ, et al. Multicenter Automatic Defibrillator Implantation Trial II Investigators. Prophylactic implantation of a defibrillator in patients with myocardial infarction and reduced ejection fraction. N Engl J Med. 2002;346:877–83.
20. Goldenberg I, Gillespie J, Moss AJ, et al. Executive Committee of the Multicenter Automatic Defibrillator Implantation Trial II. Long-term benefit of primary prevention with an implantable cardioverter-defibrillator: an extended 8-year follow-up study of the multicenter automatic defibrillator implantation trial II. Circulation. 2010;122:1265–71.
21. Bardy GH, Lee KL, Mark DB, et al. Sudden Cardiac Death in Heart Failure (SCD-HeFT) Investigators. Amiodarone or an implantable cardioverter-defibrillator for congestive heart failure. N Engl J Med. 2005;352:225–37.
22. Sjöblom J, Kalm T, Gadler F, et al. Efficacy of primary preventive ICD therapy in an unselected population of patients with reduced left ventricular ejection fraction. Europace. 2015;17:255–61.
23. Kinch Westerdahl A, Sjöblom J, Mattiasson AC, Rosenqvist M, Frykman V. Implantable cardioverter-defibrillator therapy before death. High risk for painful shocks at end of life. Circulation. 2014;129:422–9.
24. Gasparini M, Proclemer A, Klersy C, et al. Effect of long-detection interval vs standard-detection interval for implantable cardioverter-defibrillators on antitachycardia pacing and shock delivery: the ADVANCE III randomized clinical trial. JAMA. 2013;309:1903–11.
25. Lang S, Becker R, Wilke S, Hartmann M, Herzog W, Lowe B. Anxiety disorders in patients with implantable cardioverter defibrillators: frequency, course, predictors, and patients' requests for treatment. Pacing Clin Electrophysiol. 2014;37:35–47.
26. Tripp C, Huber NL, Kuhl EA, Sears SF. Measuring ICD shock anxiety: status update on the Florida Shock Anxiety Scale after over a decade of use. Pacing Clin Electrophysiol. 2019;42:1294–301.
27. Goldstein NE, Lampert R, Bradley E, Lynna J, Krumholz HM. Management of implantable cardioverter defibrillator in end-of-life care. Ann Intern Med. 2004;141:835–8.
28. Goldstein N, Carlson M, Livote E, Kutner JS. Management of implantable cardioverter defibrillators in hospice: a nationwide survey. Ann Intern Med. 2010;152:296–9.
29. Sherazi S, McNitt S, Aktas MK, et al. End-of-life care in patients with implantable cardioverter defibrillators: a MADIT-II substudy. Pacing Clin Electrophysiol. 2013;36:1273–9.
30. Waterhouse E, Ahmad F. Do implantable cardioverter defibrillators complicate end-of-life care for those with heart failure? Curr Opin Support Palliat Care. 2011;5:307–11.
31. Zellner R, Auliso MP, Lewis R. Should implantable cardioverter-defibrillators and permanent pacemakers in patients with terminal illness be deactivated? Deactivating permanent pacemaker in patients with terminal illness. Patient autonomy is paramount. Circ Arrhythm Electrophysiol. 2009;2:340–4.
32. Kramer D, Mitchell SL, Brock DW. Deactivation of pacemakers and implantable cardioverter defibrillators. Prog Cardiovasc Dis. 2012;55:290–9.

33. Kirkpatrick JN, Gottlieb M, Sehgal P, Patel R, Verdino R. Deactivation of implantable cardioverter defibrillators in terminal illness and end of life care. Am J Cardiol. 2012;109:91–4.
34. Sulmasy DP. Within you/without you: biotechnology, ontology and ethics. J Gen Intern Med. 2008;23(Suppl 1):69–72.
35. Sulmasy D, Courtois M. Unlike diamonds, defibrillators aren't forever: why it is sometimes ethical to deactivate cardiac implantable electrical devices. Camb Q Healthc Ethics. 2019;28:338–46.
36. Karches K, Sulmasy DP. Ethical considerations for a turning off pacemakers and defibrillators. Cardiac Electrophysiol Clin. 2015;7:547–55.
37. Downar J, Delaney JW, Hawryluck L, Kenny L. Guidelines for the withdrawal of life-sustaining measures. Intensive Care Med. 2016;42:1003–17.
38. Beauchamp TL, Childress JF. Principles of biomedical ethics. 7th ed. Oxford University Press, Oxford; 2012.
39. Evangelium Vitae-Gospel of Life. Encyclical Letter. John Paul II, Libreria Editrice Vaticana; 1995.
40. Khera R, Pandey A, Link MS, Sulistio MS. Managing implantable cardioverter-defibrillators at end-of-life: practical challenges and care considerations. Am J Med Sci. 2019;357:143–50.
41. Caulley L, Gillick MR, Lehmann LS. Substitute decision making in end-of-life care. N Engl J Med. 2018;378:2339–41.
42. Lampert R. Unilateral ICD deactivation: no ethical leg to stand on. Pacing Clin Electrophysiol. 2015;38:914–6.
43. Steiner JM, Patton KK, Prutkin JM, Kirkpatrick JN. Moral distress at the end of a life: when family and clinicians do not agree on implantable cardioverter-defibrillator deactivation. J Pain Symptom Manag. 2018;55:530–4.
44. Wright GA, Klein GJ, Gula LJ. Ethical and legal perspective of implantable cardioverter defibrillator deactivation or implantable cardioverter defibrillator generator replacement in the elderly. Curr Opin Cardiol. 2013;28:43–9.
45. Ruwald MH, Ruwald AC, Johansen JB, et al. Incidence of appropriate implantable cardioverter-defibrillator therapy and mortality after implantable cardioverter-defibrillator generator replacement: results from a real-world nationwide cohort. Europace. 2019:pii: euz121. https://doi.org/10.1093/europace/euz121.
46. Artico J, Ceolin R, Franco S, et al. ICD replacement in patients with intermediate left ventricular dysfunction under optimal medical treatment. Int J Cardiol. 2019;293:119–24.
47. Thompson JH, Thylén I, Moser DK. Shared decision-making about end-of-life care scenarios compared among implantable cardioverter defibrillator patients: a national cohort study. Circ Heart Fail. 2019;12:e005619. https://doi.org/10.1161/CIRCHEARTFAILURE.118.005619.
48. Goldstein N, Mehta D, Siddiqui S, et al. "That's like an act of suicide". Patients' attitudes toward deactivation of implantable defibrillators. J Gen Intern Med. 2008;23(Suppl 1):7–12.
49. Allen LA, Yager JE, Jonsson Funk M, Levy WC, Tulsky JA. Discordance between patient-predicted and model-predicted life expectancy among ambulatory patients with heart failure. JAMA. 2008;299:253342.
50. Hadler RA, Goldstein NE, Bekelman DB, et al. "Why would I choose death?": a qualitative study of patient understanding of the role and limitations of cardiac devices. J Cardiovasc Nurs. 2019;34:275–82.
51. Stewart G, Weintraub J, Pratibhu P, et al. Patient expectations from implantable defibrillators to prevent death in heart failure. J Card Fail. 2010;16:106–13.
52. Tajouri T, Ottenberg A, Hayes D, Mueller P. The use of advance directives among patients with implantable cardioverter defibrillators. Pacing Clin Electrophysiol. 2012;35:567–73.
53. Kramer DB, Kesselheim AS, Salberg L, Brock DW, Maisel WH. Ethical and legal views regarding deactivation of cardiac implantable electrical devices in patients with hypertrophic cardiomyopathy. Am J Cardiol. 2011;107:1071–5.
54. Strömberg A, Fluur C, Miller J, et al. ICD recipients' understanding of ethical issues, ICD function, and practical consequences of withdrawing the ICD in the end-of-life. Pacing Clin Electrophysiol. 2014;37:834–42.

55. Buchhalter LC, Ottenberg A, Webster TL, Swetz KM, Hayes DL, Mueller PS. Features and outcomes of patients who underwent cardiac device deactivation. JAMA Intern Med. 2014;174:80–5.

56. Trussler A, Alexander B, Campbell D, et al. Deactivation of implantable cardioverter defibrillator in patients with terminal diagnoses. Am J Cardiol. 2019;124:1064–8.

57. Raphael CE, Koa-Wing M, Stain N, Wright I, Francis DP, Kanagaratnam P. Implantable cardioverter-defibrillator recipient attitudes towards device deactivation: how much do patients want to know? Pacing Clin Electrophysiol. 2011;34:1628–33.

58. Thylen I, Moser D, Chung M, Miller J, Fluur C, Stromberg A. Are ICD recipients able to foresee if they want to withdraw therapy or deactivate defibrillator shocks? Int J Cardiol Heart Vessels. 2013;1:22–31.

59. Pedersen SS, Chaitsing R, Szili-Torok T, Jordaens L, Theuns DA. Patients' perspective on deactivation of the implantable cardioverter-defibrillator near the end of life. Am J Cardiol. 2013;111:1443–7.

60. Goldstein NE, Mather H, McKendrick K, et al. Improving communication in heart failure patient care. J Am Coll Cardiol. 2019;74:1682–92.

61. Thylén I, Moser DK, Strömberg A. Octo- and nonagenarians' outlook on life and death when living with an implantable cardioverter defibrillator: a cross-sectional study. BMC Geriatr. 2018;18:250. https://doi.org/10.1186/s12877-018-0942-9.

62. Stoevelaar R, Brinkman-Stoppelenburg A, van Driel AG, et al. Trends in time in the management of the implantable cardioverter defibrillator in the last phase of life: a retrospective study of medical records. Eur J Cardiovasc Nurs. 2019;18:449–57.

63. Pedersen SF, Knudsen C, Dilling K, Sandgaard NCF, Johansen JB. Living with an implantable cardioverter defibrillator: patients' preferences and needs for information provision and care options. Europace. 2017;19:983–90.

64. Goldstein NE, Mehta D, Teitelbaum E, Bradley EH, Morrison RS. "It's like crossing a bridge" complexities preventing physicians from discussing deactivation of implantable defibrillators at the end of life. J Gen Intern Med. 2008;23(Suppl 1):2–6.

65. Merchant FM, Binney Z, Patel A, Li J, Peddareddy LP, El-Chami MF, Leon AR, et al. Prevalence, predictors, and outcomes of advance directives in implantable cardioverter-defibrillator recipients. Heart Rhythm. 2017;14:830–6.

66. Kelley AS, Reid C, Miller D, Fins J, Lachs M. Implantable cardioverter-defibrillator deactivation at the end of life: a physician survey. Am Heart J. 2009;157:702–8.

67. Mueller PS, Jenkins SM, Bramstedt KA, Hayes DL. Deactivating implanted cardiac devices in terminally ill patients: practices and attitudes. Pacing Clin Electrophysiol. 2008;31:560–8.

68. Sherazi S, Daubert JP, Block RC, Jeevanantham V, Abdel-Gadir K, DiSalle MR. Physicians' preferences and attitudes about end-of-life care in patients with an implantable cardioverter-defibrillator. Mayo Clin Proc. 2008;83:1139–41.

69. Marinskis G, Van Erven L, Scientific Initiatives Committee EHRA. Deactivation of implantable cardioverter-defibrillators at the end of life: results of the EHRA survey. Europace. 2010;12:1176–7.

70. Bradley A, Marks A. Clinician attitudes regarding ICD deactivation in DNR/DNI patients. J Hosp Med. 2017;12:498–502.

71. Choi DY, Wagner MP, Yum B, Jannat-Khah DP, Mazique DC, Crossman DJ, et al. Improving implantable cardioverter defibrillator deactivation discussions in admitted patients made DNR and comfort care. BMJ Open Qual. 2019 Dec 4;8(4):e000730. https://doi.org/10.1136/bmjoq-2019-000730.

72. Kwok IB, Mather H, McKendrick K, Gelfman L, Hutchinson MD, Lampert RJ, et al. Evaluation of a novel educational intervention to improve conversations about implantable cardioverter-defibrillators management in patients with advanced heart failure. J Palliat Med. 2020; https://doi.org/10.1089/jpm.2020.0022.

73. Kramer D, Ottenberg A, Gerhardson S, et al. "Just because we can doesn't mean we should": views of nurses on deactivation of pacemakers and implantable cardioverter-defibrillators. J Interv Card Electrophysiol. 2011;32:243–52.

74. Hill L, McIlfatrick S, Taylor BJ, et al. Patient and professional factors that impact the perceived likelihood and confidence of healthcare professionals to discuss implantable cardioverter defibrillator deactivation in advanced heart failure: results from an international factorial survey. J Cardiovasc Nurs. 2018;33:527–35.
75. Mueller PS, Ottenberg AL, Hayes DL, Koenig BA. "I felt like the angel of death": role conflicts and moral distress among allied professionals employed by the US cardiovascular implantable electronic device industry. J Interv Card Electrophysiol. 2011;32:253–61.
76. Pilkington BC. Treating or killing? The divergent moral implications of cardiac device deactivation. J Med Philos. 2020;45(1):28–41.
77. Huddle T, Bailey FA. Pacemaker deactivation: withdrawal of support or active ending of life? Theor Med Bioeth. 2012;33:421–33.
78. Legge 22 dicembre 2017, n. 219. Norme in materia di consenso informato e di disposizioni anticipate di trattamento. Gazzetta Ufficiale Serie Generale—n. 12. 16 gennaio; 2018.
79. Turner S, Torabi S, Stilos K. Quality dying: An approach to ICD deactivation in the hospital setting. Am J Hosp Palliat Care. 2020;4:1049909120905254. https://doi.org/10.1177/1049909120905254.
80. Morgenweck CJ. Ethical considerations for discontinuing pacemakers and automatic implantable cardiac defibrillators at the end-of-life. Curr Opin Anaesthesiol. 2013;26:171–5.
81. Mueller P, Hook CC. Technological and treatment imperatives, life-sustaining technologies, and associated ethical and social challenges. Mayo Clin Proc. 2013;88:641–4.
82. Pellegrino ED. Decisions to withdraw life-sustaining treatment: a moral algorithm. JAMA. 2000;283:1065–7.
83. Schneiderman LJ. Defining medical futility and improving medical care. Bioeth Inq. 2011;8:123–31.

Withdrawal of Mechanical Circulatory Support in the Cardiac Intensive Care Unit

8

Shunichi Nakagawa, Paolo C. Colombo, and A. Reshad Garan

8.1 Introduction

As a result of advancements in healthcare technologies, many patients who suffer from severe cardiopulmonary disease can be artificially supported by life-sustaining treatment (LST) to ensure adequate oxygenation, ventilation, and cardiac output. However, it should be recognized that those LSTs can support hemodynamics temporarily, but cannot reverse the disease progression. Despite the advancement of the technology, cardiovascular disease remains the top cause of death globally, representing 31% of all global death [1]. The mortality in the intensive care unit (ICU) remains high; approximately 20% of deaths in the United States occur in an intensive care setting [2]. When treatment options are negotiated for the patients who are at their end of life (EOL) in the ICU, decision-making regarding withdrawal of LST (e.g., mechanical ventilation, vasopressor medications, and renal replacement therapy) is always challenging. Especially, in the cardiac ICU, patients are more likely to have cardiovascular implantable electronic devices (CIEDs) such as permanent pacemakers (PPM) including cardiac resynchronization therapy (CRT) and implantable cardioverter-defibrillators (ICD); more recently, they are likely to be

S. Nakagawa (✉)
Department of Medicine, Adult Palliative Care, Columbia University Irving Medical Center, New York, NY, USA
e-mail: sn2573@cumc.columbia.edu

P. C. Colombo
Department of Medicine, Division of Cardiology, Columbia University Irving Medical Center, New York, NY, USA
e-mail: pcc2001@cumc.columbia.edu

A. R. Garan
Department of Medicine, Division of Cardiology, Beth Israel Deaconess Medical Center and Harvard Medical School, Boston, MA, USA
e-mail: agaran@bidmc.harvard.edu

© The Author(s), under exclusive license to Springer Nature Switzerland AG 2021
M. Romanò (ed.), *Palliative Care in Cardiac Intensive Care Units*,
https://doi.org/10.1007/978-3-030-80112-0_8

supported by mechanical circulatory support devices (MCSDs) which include intra-aortic balloon pump (IABP), percutaneous ventricular assist devices (e.g., Impella [Abiomed, Danvers, MA] and TandemHeart [LivaNova, Pittsburgh, PA]), extracorporeal membrane oxygenation (ECMO), and durable left ventricular assist device (LVAD). Deactivation or removal of CIEDs and MCSDs at EOL poses substantial challenges to the clinician. The aim of this chapter is to highlight these challenges and provide guidance for clinicians through this process of withdrawal of LST, including CIEDs and MCSDs.

8.2 Why Is LST Withdrawal Challenging?

The withdrawal of LSTs may generate significant distress for patients, family, and even clinicians. The majority of physicians have experience with discontinuation of mechanical ventilation [3, 4] because it is more frequently encountered. However, physicians have less experience and comfort with discussing cessation of CIEDs [3, 5], and this discomfort is often increased when the patient's hemodynamics are dependent on these devices. In a survey of Heart Rhythm Society members who are experienced with CIEDs, significantly more respondents reported that they were comfortable deactivating an ICD than a PPM [6]. Similarly, significantly more medical professionals view PPM withdrawal in a PPM-dependent patient akin to physician-assisted suicide or euthanasia, while there were no differences in attitudes in the withdrawal in the non-PPM-dependent patient [7]. Furthermore, some clinicians familiar with LVADs regard withdrawing LVAD support as a form of euthanasia and feel uncomfortable turning off the device [8]. This discomfort and lack of understanding are likely among the main reasons for the fact that conversations regarding device deactivation infrequently occur at the time of initiation of these treatments [9].

Communication regarding the EOL experience at an earlier stage is paramount. In LVAD therapy, for example, it has been proposed that the medical team should have a thorough conversation with patients and family prior to LVAD implantation as "preparedness planning" [10]. However, this process has not been standardized yet and there is great variability between LVAD institutions. As a result, bereaved caregivers of LVAD patients describe a high level of confusion at the EOL [11]. Similarly, in other LSTs too, the lack of communication results in a great deal of confusion and distress on the patient side at the EOL [12–14]. This discomfort is likely caused by the fact that death may quickly ensue after the withdrawal of MCSDs.

With MCSDs, in particular, forethought with respect to the patient's disease trajectory is often encouraged to avoid a "bridge to nowhere" situation. Such a situation occurs when MCSDs are placed initially for rapidly progressive circulatory collapse with the hope for the recovery or more long-term future treatment such as cardiac transplant or long-term durable LVADs, but none of these options are ultimately available due to the medical condition. In this situation, MCSDs continue to support the patient's circulation but only in the ICU setting. This scenario where the patient is confined to the ICU for the rest of her or his life may be emotionally charged and can be made more challenging if the patient is awake and aware of their dependence on the device.

8.3   Ethical Consideration in Withdrawal of Cardiopulmonary Devices

One reason for clinician discomfort with LST withdrawal is confusion between euthanasia or physician-assisted suicide and withdrawal of LSTs. Euthanasia is defined as an act that intentionally causes death in someone who is very sick or suffering. In physician-assisted suicide, a physician helps a patient in taking her or his own life by intentionally providing a lethal dose of medication with the knowledge that the patient might commit suicide [15]. As shown in Table 8.1, there is a clear distinction between withdrawal of LST and euthanasia/physician-assisted suicide in terms of physician's intent and cause of death [16].

It has been generally accepted, both ethically and legally, that patients have a right to refuse any treatments or request withdrawal of any therapy as long as the burden of the treatment outweighs the benefits [17–20]. There is no legal or ethical distinction among the type of LSTs, regardless of the dependence on those treatments, such as CIEDs or MCSDs [16, 21, 22].

When withdrawal of LSTs is considered, clinicians should consider several questions: (1) Who is making decisions for the patient? (2) By what criteria are those decisions being made? (3) How are conflicts among decision-makers prevented or resolved? [18] The decision should be made by the patient when he or she has a clear decision-making capacity, and by a surrogate when the patient is incapacitated. Each patient is unique and weighs benefits and burdens differently with their own values, preferences, and healthcare goals. Ultimately, the patients' decisions have priority over clinicians' decisions and clinicians should not impose their moral views on patients [16]. Often there are conflicts among the patient, family, and clinicians. In many instances, these may stem from misunderstanding or miscommunication regarding the goals of care and/or the role of LSTs.

In such situations, palliative care teams may be particularly helpful because this discussion requires sensitive communication among patients, families, and the interdisciplinary care team. If necessary, consultation from the ethics team, social work, or chaplain should be used proactively. If clinicians feel uncomfortable with the withdrawal of LSTs for emotional or moral reasons (which may be more common in a "bridge to nowhere" situation), they should not be compelled to join the

Table 8.1 The difference between withdrawal of LST and physician-assisted suicide/euthanasia

	Withdrawal of LST	Physician-assisted suicide, euthanasia
Physician's intent	Remove the burdensome treatment	Terminate the life
Cause of death	The underlying disease	Intervention provided

deactivation process [23]. However, they should not abandon the patient and they should facilitate the transfer of care to another clinician who is willing to help the patient [24].

8.4   Approach to Specific Life-Sustaining Treatments

Removal or deactivation of different forms of LST including mechanical ventilation, ICD, PPM, and MCSDs (IABP, pVAD, ECMO, and durable LVAD) has unique considerations. Since withdrawal of mechanical ventilation is one of the most commonly accepted practices, aspects of this practice may be applied to withdrawal of other devices as well.

8.5   Mechanical Ventilation

The most common approaches to withdrawing ventilator support are immediate extubation (removal of the endotracheal tube or discontinuation of ventilator support in patients with tracheostomy) and terminal weaning (gradual reduction of inspired oxygen concentration and/or mandatory ventilator rate). Both of these approaches are supported by guidelines from major medical societies [25–27]. The patient's and clinician's comfort, and the family's perceptions, should influence the manner in which withdrawal is pursued. Even though a decision has been made to withdraw life support, such a decision is often emotionally charged. It is paramount for clinicians to focus on the comfort of the patient and provide guidance and support to family at each step of the way. Below is the checklist for the withdrawal process [28–30].

After extubation, clinicians should monitor the patient's condition carefully. The only way to monitor the degree of comfort or discomfort is serial physical examinations at the bedside. Diagnostic testing or other methods of monitoring the patient should not be pursued. Because patients often cannot express themselves during this process, clinicians should make clinical management decisions using nonverbal cues, such as facial expressions, rate and pattern of breathing, use of accessory muscles, and movement of the body.

8.6   MCSDs (IABP, Impella, ECMO, and LVAD)

As opposed to mechanical ventilation, a smaller group of healthcare providers has experience and comfort with deactivation or withdrawal of MCSDs; this may be related to the fact that patients are not only hemodynamically dependent on MCSDs but they may also be alert and involved in discussions regarding the process of MCSD withdrawal. The process of withdrawal of MCSDs is akin to that of mechanical ventilation (Table 8.2), but clinicians should acknowledge that survival after deactivation of MCSDs could be very short; although it could be hours to a few days

Table 8.2 The flow of withdrawal of mechanical ventilation

6–12 h prior to extubation
1. Stop artificial nutrition (enteral feeding). Start anticholinergic to reduce airway secretions.
Immediately prior to extubation
1. Encourage family to make arrangements for special music or rituals.
2. Explain the process of withdrawal and counsel on potential outcomes following withdrawal. Clarify if family would like to be present in the room during the withdrawal process.
3. When there are multiple LSTs (renal replacement therapy, vasopressors, ICDs, etc.), consider the order of withdrawal and share the strategy among the medical team.
4. Document clinical findings, discussion with patients or surrogates, and goals of care. DNR and DNI order should be confirmed and documented. If necessary, contact the appropriate department in the hospital to acquire authorization.
5. Ensure that all the alarms are turned off. Instruct respiratory therapy and nursing staffs their roles.
6. Remove restraints and unnecessary medical paraphernalia.
During extubation
1. Make sure that paralytics have worn off, if they have been used.
2. Administer anticholinergic to reduce secretions (20–30 min in case glycopyrrolate 0.2–0.4 mg IV, several hours in case of scopolamine patch).
3. Administer an IV bolus of opioid (e.g., morphine 2–10 mg IV) for shortness of breath and a benzodiazepine (e.g., lorazepam 1–2 mg IV) for anxiety 10–15 min prior to the extubation. Titrate medications to control labored breathing and achieve the desired state of sedation prior to extubation.
Consider an IV continuous infusion of opioid +/− benzodiazepine.
4. Anticipate that an additional dose of opioid or benzodiazepine may be needed before withdrawal. Have a syringe of additional opioid or benzodiazepine ready to administer at bedside.
After extubation
1. If distress is noted, utilize additional bolus doses of opioids (e.g., morphine 5–10 mg IV push q 10min and/or benzodiazepines (e.g., lorazepam 1–2 mg IV push q10min) until distress is relieved. Infusion rates can be increased, but change in the infusion rates will have a delayed effect.
2. Be prepared to spend additional time at bedside to ensure adequate symptom management. Specific dosage is less important than the goal of symptom relief. A goal should be to keep respiratory rate <30 and eliminate grimacing, agitation, and labored respirations.
3. After death occurs, encourage the family to spend as much time at bedside as they require; provide acute grief support and follow-up bereavement support.

[21], most often it is in the range of minutes [31]. Therefore, the following two points should be emphasized.

First, the deactivation process should be clearly outlined among the medical team. More frequently, patients are on other types of LSTs as well (mechanical ventilation, renal replacement therapy, vasopressors, etc.) and those should be discontinued at the same time as MCSD deactivation. If the family requests "the most natural death with dignity," for example, it may be prudent to withdraw mechanical ventilation first prior to the MCSD as the patient could otherwise be still connected to the ventilator at the time of death.

Second, clinicians should take into account that circulation will diminish after MCSDs are deactivated and it will take more time for the medications to take effect if distress is noted [32]. Therefore, enough comfort medications including opioid and benzodiazepine should be given prior to deactivation, in order to achieve optimal symptom management during the potentially short dying process.

Cardiac ICU team should maintain close communication with a person who is familiar with that specific MCSD prior to the deactivation, such as a perfusionist or an LVAD nurse practitioner, in order to learn the specifics of device management. It is strongly recommended that such members of the healthcare team join the actual deactivation process to help silencing any device alarms and/or turning off the MCSD.

8.7　The Role of Palliative Care Consultation

Palliative care consultation has been recommended in the setting of cardiogenic shock, though the optimal timing of consultation remains incompletely defined [33]. In a study of patients supported by VA-ECMO who ultimately underwent device withdrawal, early palliative care consultation was associated with a shorter length of time (7.6 vs. 13.5 days) of ECMO support prior to death [34]. However, it is important to recognize that due to a relative lack of formally trained palliative care specialists, non-palliative care specialists providing care in the ICU should be encouraged to have familiarity with the practice of palliative care to ensure that important needs of the patient and family are addressed for patients with cardiogenic shock supported by MCSDs [35].

Importantly, anticipatory guidance may impact the experience of MCSD deactivation positively. Among a cohort of durable LVAD recipients, a subset of patients were capable of articulating an "unacceptable condition" prior to device implantation during routine preoperative palliative care consultation. While the ability to articulate an unacceptable condition did not impact the decision to deactivate the durable LVAD, those who articulated the unacceptable condition were less likely to expire in an ICU and less likely to require an ethics consultation prior to their death [36].

8.8　Conclusion

As the use of MCSDs increases in the care of patients with cardiogenic shock, healthcare providers will increasingly be confronted with issues surrounding the withdrawal of these devices. It is important that clinicians understand the differences between MCSD withdrawal and physician-assisted suicide or euthanasia. Careful planning by the medical team regarding the process of device deactivation or withdrawal is critical in ensuring a dignified death for the patient. Palliative care consultation early in the course of cardiogenic shock should be utilized when available for anticipatory guidance in the event that MCSD withdrawal is pursued. When

MCSDs are implanted electively as in the case of durable LVADs, clinicians should address the concept of "unacceptable condition" that facilitates end-of-life care when necessary.

References

1. https://www.who.int/news-room/fact-sheets/detail/cardiovascular-diseases-(cvds). Accessed December 2020.
2. Angus DC, Barnato AE, Linde-Zwirble WT, Weissfeld LA, Watson RS, Rickert T, et al. Use of intensive care at the end of life in the United States: an epidemiologic study. Crit Care Med. 2004;32(3):638–43.
3. Kramer DB, Kesselheim AS, Brock DW, Maisel WH. Ethical and legal views of physicians regarding deactivation of cardiac implantable electrical devices: a quantitative assessment. Heart Rhythm. 2010;7(11):1537–42.
4. Faber-Langendoen K. The clinical management of dying patients receiving mechanical ventilation. A survey of physician practice. Chest. 1994;106(3):880–8.
5. Goldstein N, Bradley E, Zeidman J, Mehta D, Morrison RS. Barriers to conversations about deactivation of implantable defibrillators in seriously ill patients: results of a nationwide survey comparing cardiology specialists to primary care physicians. J Am Coll Cardiol. 2009;54(4):371–3.
6. Mueller PS, Jenkins SM, Bramstedt KA, Hayes DL. Deactivating implanted cardiac devices in terminally ill patients: practices and attitudes. Pacing Clin Electrophysiol. 2008;31(5):560–8.
7. Kapa S, Mueller PS, Hayes DL, Asirvatham SJ. Perspectives on withdrawing pacemaker and implantable cardioverter-defibrillator therapies at end of life: results of a survey of medical and legal professionals and patients. Mayo Clin Proc. 2010;85(11):981–90.
8. Swetz KM, Cook KE, Ottenberg AL, Chang N, Mueller PS. Clinicians' attitudes regarding withdrawal of left ventricular assist devices in patients approaching the end of life. Eur J Heart Fail. 2013;15(11):1262–6.
9. Goldstein NE, Mehta D, Teitelbaum E, Bradley EH, Morrison RS. "It's like crossing a bridge" complexities preventing physicians from discussing deactivation of implantable defibrillators at the end of life. J Gen Intern Med. 2008;23(Suppl 1):2–6.
10. Swetz KM, Kamal AH, Matlock DD, Dose AM, Borkenhagen LS, Kimeu AK, et al. Preparedness planning before mechanical circulatory support: a "how-to" guide for palliative medicine clinicians. J Pain Symptom Manag. 2014;47(5):926–35. e6
11. McIlvennan CK, Jones J, Allen LA, Swetz KM, Nowels C, Matlock DD. Bereaved caregiver perspectives on the end-of-life experience of patients with a left ventricular assist device. JAMA Intern Med. 2016;176(4):534–9.
12. McIlvennan CK, Allen LA. Palliative care in patients with heart failure. BMJ. 2016;353:i1010.
13. Goldstein NE, Mehta D, Siddiqui S, Teitelbaum E, Zeidman J, Singson M, et al. "That's like an act of suicide" patients' attitudes toward deactivation of implantable defibrillators. J Gen Intern Med. 2008;23(Suppl 1):7–12.
14. Butler K. Knocking on heaven's door : the path to a better way of death. First Scribner hardcover edition. Ed. New York: Scribner; 2013.
15. Beauchamp TL, Childress JF. Principles of biomedical ethics. 7th ed. New York: Oxford University Press; 2013.
16. Lampert R, Hayes DL, Annas GJ, Farley MA, Goldstein NE, Hamilton RM, et al. HRS expert consensus statement on the management of cardiovascular implantable electronic devices (CIEDs) in patients nearing end of life or requesting withdrawal of therapy. Heart Rhythm. 2010;7(7):1008–26.
17. Pellegrino ED. Is it ethical to withdraw low-burden interventions in chronically ill patients? JAMA. 2000;284(11):1380–2.

18. Pellegrino ED. Decisions to withdraw life-sustaining treatment: a moral algorithm. JAMA. 2000;283(8):1065–7.
19. Snyder L, Leffler C. Ethics, human rights committee ACoP. Ethics manual: fifth edition. Ann Intern Med. 2005;142(7):560–82.
20. McIlvennan CK, Swetz KM. Lack of agreement with what we think is right does not necessarily equal an ethical problem: respecting patients' goals of care. Am J Bioeth. 2016;16(8):13–5.
21. Brush S, Budge D, Alharethi R, McCormick AJ, MacPherson JE, Reid BB, et al. End-of-life decision making and implementation in recipients of a destination left ventricular assist device. J Heart Lung Transplant. 2010;29(12):1337–41.
22. Swetz KM, Freeman MR, Mueller PS, Park SJ. Clinical management of continuous-flow left ventricular assist devices in advanced heart failure. J Heart Lung Transplant. 2010;29(9):1081.
23. Zellner RA, Aulisio MP, Lewis WR. Should implantable cardioverter-defibrillators and permanent pacemakers in patients with terminal illness be deactivated? Deactivating permanent pacemaker in patients with terminal illness. Patient autonomy is paramount. Circ Arrhythm Electrophysiol. 2009;2(3):340–4.
24. Mueller PS, Hook CC, Hayes DL, editors. Ethical analysis of withdrawal of pacemaker or implantable cardioverter-defibrillator support at the end of life. Mayo Clin Proc. 2003;78(8):959–63.
25. Downar J, Delaney JW, Hawryluck L, Kenny L. Guidelines for the withdrawal of life-sustaining measures. Intensive Care Med. 2016;42(6):1003–17.
26. Truog RD, Campbell ML, Curtis JR, Haas CE, Luce JM, Rubenfeld GD, et al. Recommendations for end-of-life care in the intensive care unit: a consensus statement by the American College of Critical Care Medicine. Crit Car Med. 2008;36(3):953–63.
27. Lanken PN, Terry PB, DeLisser HM, Fahy BF, Hansen-Flaschen J, Heffner JE, et al. An official American Thoracic Society clinical policy statement: palliative care for patients with respiratory diseases and critical illnesses. Am J Resp Crit Care Med. 2008;177(8):912–27.
28. von Gunten C, Weissman DE. Ventilator withdrawal protocol. J Palliat Med. 2003;6(5):773–4.
29. von Gunten C, Weissman DE. Symptom control for ventilator withdrawal in the dying patient. J Palliat Med. 2003;6(5):774–5.
30. von Gunten C, Weissman DE. Information for patients and families about ventilator withdrawal. J Palliat Med. 2003;6(5):775–6.
31. Dunlay SM, Strand JJ, Wordingham SE, Stulak JM, Luckhardt AJ, Swetz KM. Dying with a left ventricular assist device as destination therapy. Circ Heart Fail. 2016;9(10):e003096.
32. Gafford EF, Luckhardt AJ, Swetz KM. Deactivation of a left ventricular assist device at the end of life. J Palliat Med. 2013;16(8):980–2.
33. van Diepen S, Katz JN, Albert NM, et al. Contemporary management of cardiogenic shock: a scientific statement from the American Heart Association. Circulation. 2017;136(16):e232–68.
34. Godfrey S, Sahoo A, Sanchez J, et al. The role of palliative care in withdrawal of venoarterial extracorporeal membrane oxygenation for cardiogenic shock. J Pain Symptom Manage. 2021;61:1139–46.
35. Nakagawa S, Garan AR. Hospice use and palliative care for patients with heart failure: never say never in medicine, but it is never too early to start the conversation. JAMA Cardiol. 2018;3(10):926–8.
36. Nakagawa S, Takayama H, Takeda K, et al. Association between "Unacceptable Condition" expressed in palliative care consultation before left ventricular assist device implantation and care received at the end of life. J Pain Symptom Manage. 2020;60(5):976–983.e1.

Do-Not-Attempt-Resuscitation Orders in the Cardiac Intensive Care Unit

9

Susanna Price

9.1 Cardiopulmonary Resuscitation

Closed chest massage and defibrillation were introduced in the 1960s as an intervention for patients with ventricular fibrillation, usually in the context of acute myocardial infarction, from which they would otherwise have been expected to make a good recovery [1]. As awareness of cardiopulmonary resuscitation (CPR) has increased, it has expanded such that it is the default option for every patient admitted to hospital unless a decision to not attempt resuscitation has been made, and an order signed to that effect (do not attempt resuscitation (DNAR)/cardiopulmonary resuscitation (DNACPR)).

In a landmark court case [2] where the presence of a DNACPR order without patient/family discussion was challenged, the sheer physicality of CPR was described: 'a violent and invasive physical treatment used to attempt to maintain the circulation and breathing of a person whose heartbeat and/or breathing has stopped (cardiorespiratory arrest) and to restart the heart if possible. It involves repeated, forceful compression of the bare chest to a depth of 5–6 centimetres at a compression rate of 100–120 per minute (this is so intensive that someone giving chest compressions will become fatigued within 2 minutes), attempted inflation of the lungs by forcing air or oxygen into the lungs, often through a tube inserted into a patient's windpipe, the injection of drugs into veins or into bones and the delivery of high-voltage electric shocks (defibrillation) across the bare chest'.

Cardiorespiratory arrest is an integral part of the natural process of dying from any cause. Application of CPR is no longer limited to patients with myocardial infarction and ventricular fibrillation, and unfortunately may include circumstances

S. Price (✉)
Consultant Cardiologist & Intensivist, Royal Brompton Hospital, London, UK

National Heart & Lung Institute, Imperial College, London, UK
e-mail: S.Price@rbht.nhs.uk

© The Author(s), under exclusive license to Springer Nature
Switzerland AG 2021
M. Romanò (ed.), *Palliative Care in Cardiac Intensive Care Units*,
https://doi.org/10.1007/978-3-030-80112-0_9

in which patients may be critically ill and in which in the event of cardiac arrest, CPR either would not work (whilst subjecting them to violent physical treatment at the end of their life and depriving them of a dignified death) or may restore cardiac function only briefly, thereby prolonging their period of suffering from their underlying terminal illness. As the complexity of patients admitted to the CICU increases [3], the relevance of discussions around resuscitation becomes evermore pertinent.

9.2 Intensive Care Medicine: A Balance of Risks and Benefits

Cardiac intensive care is concerned with the treatment of the most critically ill cardiac patients with, at risk of or recovering from potentially life-threatening failure of the heart and other organ systems. It aims to provide organ system support and investigate, diagnose and treat critical illness, with the aim of restoring patients to a high quality of life. A vital part of an intensive care clinician's role is to weigh risks and benefits of every single intervention in an attempt to steer the patient through their critical illness so they survive, and survive well. In doing so, it is important to avoid interventions that may cause suffering with no realistic chance of benefit, including CPR in certain patients. The challenge is to predict which patients will benefit.

The outcome following cardiac arrest is critically dependent on a number of factors including the patient's age, underlying diagnosis and comorbidities, cause of cardiorespiratory arrest and rapidity of initiation and quality of CPR. Considering outcomes from cardiac arrest in the ICU setting (ICU-CA) numerous challenges exist. First, there are limited data and significant variation in the incidence of ICU-CA. Second, the patients admitted to ICU are highly selected and therefore outcomes from ICU-CA are not directly comparable to the non-ICU population. Third the degree of monitoring and interventions are significantly different from the general ward, as is the medical response to cardiac arrest. These all suggest that the ICU-CA population is distinct and has different outcomes than the non-ICU patient population and this makes balancing risks and benefits and predicting outcomes particularly challenging [4]. Although relatively uncommon with a reported prevalence of 5–78 per 1000 admissions to the general ICU, outcomes vary, with reported survival to hospital discharge of 17% (95% CI: 9.5–28.5%) [5]. There are no high-quality data regarding ICU-CA in the specialist cardiac unit, but small studies suggest survival to discharge of approximately 50% [6]. The importance of the underlying disease prognosis on outcomes following CPR cannot be overstated. For example, the likelihood of a cancer patient in an ICU having successful CPR such that they recover to leave hospital has been reported at only 2.2%. When considering CICU, the underlying disease process and relative prognosis are equally important to consider, as despite advances in medical treatment cardiogenic shock remains particularly lethal, with 30-day mortality of up to 62%, and fewer than 15% of patients alive after 6 years [7]. Further, data suggest that in survivors, the prognosis and burden of symptomatology may be equivalent to or worse than many malignancies [8]. Thus, as CPR is not a benign or neutral intervention, in some patients who are actively dying despite critical care it may be judged an inappropriate intervention at the time of death. Indeed, if the heart is the final organ to fail/stop, it is probably inappropriate to attempt to restart it. In other patients the risks and benefits may need to be carefully weighed up in order to avoid inadvertent harm from CPR or failure to institute resuscitation when it would likely be of benefit.

When contemplating a resuscitation decision, the fundamental principles of medical ethics apply: autonomy, beneficence, non-maleficence and justice, although there are significant differences between countries regarding the cultural, social and economic contexts in which the decisions are made [8, 9]. These have been particularly highlighted in the 2020 COVID-19 pandemic [10].

9.3   The Utility of DNACPR Orders

Although there is wide variation between countries, historically, the decision not to institute CPR in the event of a cardiac arrest has been recorded generally on a specific form. The need for this documentation relates to the immediacy of the response required from clinicians and the resuscitation team in order for CPR to be effective in those likely to benefit, and the wish (in the interests of good medical practice) to avoid inflicting CPR on those who do not want it or are dying from irreversible conditions. In some countries a DNACPR order is required to be recorded routinely on all acute admissions.

DNACPR orders are not legally binding and may need to be revised/reversed depending on the clinical context including around the time of a specific intervention/surgery or in the event the patient recovers from a position where it seemed previously likely that they would not recover from their critical illness. DNACPR decisions should be made in emergent situations for incapacitated patients, in which case they should be discussed with the patient's representatives/next of kin at the earliest opportunity, and may well need to be revised at a later date should the patient recover. Previously clinicians were insufficiently proactive regarding reversing decisions regarding resuscitation, and for this reason, where DNACPR forms are used, they include a time limit.

A number of situations may arise where a decision has been made that CPR on the ICU would be inappropriate and a DNACPR decision may be required (Table 9.1) [2].

9.4   The Unintended Consequences of DNACPR Orders

A DNACPR order should relate to CPR alone and no other aspect of care should be impacted—however, there is evidence that it does negatively influence the likelihood of both medical and nursing interventions, including referral to critical care [11]. Additional potential downsides include that patients with a DNACPR order in place are more likely to be denied ICU admission, even if they might benefit as they

Table 9.1 Situations where a DNACPR decision may be required

Clinical context
• At the request of a person with capacity
• As an important element of end-of-life care for a person who is terminally ill from an advanced/irreversible disease
• As an element of care in someone who continues to deteriorate despite all appropriate treatment
• Where a patient has suffered a sudden, catastrophic event from which no recovery can be reasonably expected
• As an element of care of patients who are approaching the end of their lives

may 'trigger heuristic decision-making' by the intensivist [11]. There is additional evidence that if in place, patients are less likely to receive disease-modifying agents and interventions if admitted with acute heart failure [12]. Further, where a DNACPR order is present, the number of interventions by ICU nursing staff is reduced [13], and there can be a false and potentially dangerous perception amongst all staff that DNACPR is synonymous with do not treat/escalate [14].

As a DNACPR decision is one that may potentially deprive the patient of life-saving treatment, there should be a presumption of patient involvement. Indeed, not to do so has been judged to be in breach of Article 8 of the European Court of Human Rights, and clinicians must consult with patients except in limited circumstances [2]. Of note, the patient potentially finding the topic distressing is insufficient reason not to have their involvement in such important decisions about their life. Where the patient lacks capacity, best interest decisions (including DNACPR) should be discussed with those who might know their values, wishes and preferences, the patient representatives/next of kin. This discussion may extend to other life-saving treatments about which decisions have to be made, and also in the final, closing stages of life.

9.5 Shared Decision-Making

In the early days of critical care, the ethical principles of beneficence and non-maleficence supported the largely paternalistic approach of physicians in their decisions regarding who should or should not receive CPR. Increasingly the importance of patient-centred care as pivotal to high-quality healthcare is recognised, and the principle of respect for patient autonomy dominates medical practice in many countries. Despite this, much treatment that patients receive remains physician centred rather than based on the patients' preferences. In December 2010 the Salzburg Global Seminar resulted in publication of the Salzburg statement on shared decision-making [15]. In addition to the numerous benefits described, it is of note that patients involved in shared decision-making are more likely than their doctors to defer or decline interventions, but with no measurable impact on health outcomes or satisfaction. Shared decision-making is a very specific process, summarised in ten domains, and is regarded by many as the pinnacle of patient-centred care [16].

The concept of shared decision-making is supported by legislation in a number of countries and endorsed by many professional bodies. Despite the supporting evidence and widespread legal acceptance, numerous challenges exist, mainly relating to misunderstanding and lack of knowledge regarding the process by both healthcare practitioners and patients [17]. Thus, between 37% and 58% of seriously ill patients do not wish to discuss their preferences for resuscitation, and many physicians fail to raise the subject [18]. Most patients have not made an advance decision regarding resuscitation wishes, and for those who have, their decisions may be inconsistently followed and/or subject to misinterpretation by clinicians [18]. Additionally there can be a divergence of perceptions between healthcare providers and patients on the goals, benefits (including the likelihood of success of CPR) and side effects and possible complications of interventions [19].

Although the process of shared decision-making regarding resuscitation status should involve ensuring that patients and their families understand the decisions they are making, this is not always achieved, even by experienced clinicians [20]. In the ICU setting patients often have strong views regarding treatments they poorly understand, with one-quarter being unable to identify features of CPR and over one-third significantly overestimating CPR survival to hospital discharge, possibly in part related to inaccurate media portrayal. This is compounded further, in that the perception of patients, carers and medical professionals regarding prognosis in cardiac disease is inaccurate, with only 29% of patients considering heart failure to be a serious condition, and 67% believing patients with the diagnosis will live longer than those with cancer [20]. This position is made even more difficult by the poor tools available to healthcare professionals for prognostication in cardiac disease and the critically ill. All these factors make shared decision-making regarding resuscitation challenging in the critical care setting—but not impossible. The experienced medical team must be able to help the patient (or their representatives/next of kin) navigate these complexities to come to the best decision for the patient at that time, including honesty where uncertainty exists.

9.6 Moving Beyond DNACPR Towards Resuscitation Plans

The risks to a patient of having a DNACPR order in place, where it may be misinterpreted to go beyond CPR, even in a patient in the ICU and in receipt of aggressive medical interventions are clear [13]. This misinterpretation may result from a number of factors including a lack of understanding of hospital policy, and the ethical and moral values of the staff. Further, a DNACPR decision can be conflated with anticipation of imminent death and is somewhat stigmatising. As a result, a number of bodies are now recommending alternative approaches to resuscitation decisions, including replacing DNACPR orders with clearly defined treatment and resuscitation plans jointly determined by the MDT and patient (or relatives/next of kin where they lack capacity). These include advance care planning with a broader reach, including decisions around resuscitation such as the Recommended Summary Plan for Emergency Care and Treatment (ReSPECT) [21] and Physician Order for

Life-Sustaining Treatment (POLST), widely used in the USA, which encourages physicians and patients to discuss which treatments (including CPR) would be desired should the patient deteriorate [22].

The Universal Form of Treatment Options (UFTO) provides much more contextualisation than a DNACPR order, with a focus on treatments the patient would wish to have rather than those withheld. In steering clear of tick boxes, and allowing free text, it ensures less reflexive decision-making, and where used, it is completed for all inpatients, with the aim to make discussions around resuscitation more routine and reduce negative associations with any subsequent decision, as well as provide clarity for goals of care [23]. Research into use of the UFTO in combination with a leaflet ('talking to your doctor') compared with a standard DNACPR order demonstrated its use to be associated with significant reduction in medical error from inappropriately aggressive or conservative care, without change to overall mortality [23].

Resuscitation plans are not simply a new type of form, but rather reflect a cultural shift that advocates for a change in the medical approach to decisions around treatment/interventions [24]. The emphasis is on early and considered decisions, transparent and honest communication with patients (or relatives/next of kin where necessary) and delivery of medical care that is appropriate given their baseline status and prognosis, including recommendation for a conservative approach, symptom control or palliative care when required. In considering critical care without walls, the benefits of shifting from DNACPR to resuscitation plans also extend to supporting outreach teams, with a perceived ability to tailor care appropriately (including end-of-life care), increased speed in decision-making and improved communication about goals of care during medical handover [23, 25].

The language of decision-making around resuscitation is also shifting. In the US-based POLST resuscitation plan 'selective treatment' has replaced 'limited treatment' and 'comfort-focused care' has replaced 'comfort measures', intending to emphasise that specific care is given rather than care is being limited/withdrawn. Rather than DNACPR, the concept of 'allow natural death (AND)' has been introduced in some parts of the USA, where the phrase has been shown to be associated with increased frequency and acceptance of resuscitation decisions [26]. At such a key moment in a patient's life, making the best decisions for them or reassuring relatives that they are receiving the optimal care is vital. Future iterations of resuscitation plans will surely evolve to better meet the needs of optimal decision-making around CPR in the ICU setting [24].

9.7 Conclusions

Providing our critically ill cardiac patients with the treatment they deserve—based on their symptoms and prognosis rather than their diagnosis—is vital. Included in this are decisions surrounding resuscitation. The negative impact from DNACPR orders in intensive care is clear and it is evident that we need to move to a different way of discussing resuscitation with our patients. Determining an individual's wishes for future emergency care when they have the capacity to make or express choices is vital, and ideally should take place before CICU admission. Although this will take time to be universally implemented, moving towards proper shared decision-making, changing the rhetoric around resuscitation discussions and decisions away from DNACPR whilst moving towards resuscitation planning are surely the way forward. The implications for reduction in harmful treatment, unnecessary interventions and costs (to the patient, their relatives, healthcare workers and society) are clear.

References

1. Kouwenhoven WB, Jude JR, Knickerbocker GG. Closed chest cardiac massage. JAMA. 1960;173:1064–7.
2. https://www.judiciary.uk/wp-content/uploads/2014/06/tracey-approved.pdf
3. Morrow DA, Fang JC, Fintel DJ, et al. Evolution of critical care cardiology: transformation of the cardiovascular intensive care unit and the emerging need for new medical staffing and training models. Circulation. 2012;126:1408–28.
4. Cook J, Thomas M. Cardiac arrest in ICU. J Intensive Care Soc. 2017;18:173.
5. Armstrong RA, Kane C, Oglesby F, et al. The incidence of cardiac arrest in the intensive care unit: a systematic review and meta-analysis. J Intensive Care Soc. 2019;20(2):144–54.
6. Mohnle P, Huge V, Polasek J, et al. Survival after cardiac arrest and changing task profile of the cardiac arrest team in a tertiary care center. ScientificWorldJournal. 2012;2012:294512.
7. Lindholm MG, Køber L, Boesgaard S, Torp-Pedersen C, Aldershvile J, Trandolapril Cardiac Evaluation Study Group. Cardiogenic shock complicating acute myocardial infarction; prognostic impact of early and late shock development. Eur Heart J. 2003;24:258–65.
8. Price S, Haxby E. Managing futility in critically ill patients with cardiac disease. Nat Rev Cardiol. 2013;10:723–31.
9. Alexander JO, Gibbs AC, Malyon A, et al. Themes and variations: an exploratory international investigation into resuscitation decision-making. Resuscitation. 2016;103:75–81.
10. https://www.cqc.org.uk/sites/default/files/20201204%20DNACPR%20Interim%20 Report%20-%20FINAL.pdf
11. James FR, Power N, Shondipon L. Decision-making in intensive care medicine—a review. J Intensive Care Soc. 2018;19(3):247–58.
12. Chen JLT, Sosnov J, Lessard D, Goldberg RJ. Impact of do-not-resuscitation orders on quality of care performance measures in patients hospitalized with acute heart failure. Am Heart J. 2008;156:78–84.
13. Henneman EA, Baird B, Bellamy PE, Faber LL, Oye RK. Effect of do-not-resuscitate orders on the nursing care of critically ill patients. Am J Crit Care. 1994;3:467–72.
14. Fritz Z, Slowther M, Perkins G. Resuscitation policy should focus on the patient, not the decision. BMJ. 2017;356:j813.
15. Alambuya RN, Ali S, Apostolidis K, et al. Salzburg statement on shared decision making. BMJ. 2011;342:d1745. https://doi.org/10.1136/bmj.d1745.
16. White DB, Braddock CH, Bereknyei S, Curtis JR. Toward shared decision making at the end of life in intensive care units: opportunities for improvement. Arch Intern Med. 2007;167:461–7.
17. Gott M, Ingleton C, Bennett MI, Gardiner C. Transitions to palliative care in acute hospitals in England: qualitative study. BMJ. 2011;342:d1773.
18. Hofmann JC, Wenger NS, Davis RB, Teno J, Connors AF Jr, Desbiens N. Patient preferences for communication with physicians about end-of-life decisions. SUPPORT Investigators. Study to understand prognoses and preference for outcomes and risks of treatment. Ann Intern Med. 1997;127:1–12.

19. Khatcheressian J, Harrington SB, Lyckholm LJ, Smith TJ. 'Futile care': what to do when your patient insists on chemotherapy that likely won't help. Oncology (Williston Park). 2008;22:881–8.
20. Singer PA, Robertson G, Roy DJ. Bioethics for clinicians: 6. Advance care planning. CMAJ. 1996;155:1689–92.
21. Fritz Z, Pitcher D, Hawkes C, Nolan JP. Development of a national approach to resuscitation decisions: the recommended summary plan for emergency care and treatment (ReSPECT). Resuscitation. 2020;148:98–107. Epub 2020 Jan 13. https://doi.org/10.1016/j.resuscitation.2020.01.003.
22. Cantor MD. Improving advance care planning: lessons from POLST. Physician orders for life-sustaining treatment. J Am Geriatr Soc. 2000 Oct;48(10):1343–4. https://doi.org/10.1111/j.1532-5415.2000.tb02613.x.
23. Fritz Z, Malyon A, Frankau JM, et al. The Universal Form of Treatment Options (UFTO) as an alternative to Do Not Attempt Cardiopulmonary Resuscitation (DNACPR) orders: a mixed methods evaluation of the effects on clinical practice and patient care. PLoS One. 2013;8:e70977.
24. Dignam C, Brown M, Thompson CH. Moving from "do not resuscitate" orders to standardized resuscitation plans and shared decision-making in hospital inpatients. Gerontol Geriatr Med. 2021;7:23337214211003431. https://doi.org/10.1177/23337214211003431.
25. Dahill M, Powter L, Garland L, et al. Improving documentation of treatment escalation decisions in acute care. BMJ Qual Improv Rep. 2013;2:u200617.w1077.
26. Fan SY, Wang YW, Lin IM. Allow natural death versus do-not-resuscitate: titles, information contents, outcomes, and the considerations related to do-not-resuscitate decision. BMC Palliat Care. 2018;17:114.

Palliative Sedation in Cardiac Intensive Care Units: When, Why, How

10

Luciano Orsi

10.1 Introduction

In the final stages of heart diseases, symptoms such as dyspnoea, anxiety, pain, psychomotor agitation, delirium and psycho-existential suffering can intensify and become unresponsive to therapies, triggering unbearable suffering for the patient. In these circumstances, the goal of PS is to control patient suffering, relieving refractory symptoms to improve the quality of the patient's remaining life with adequate clinical and interpersonal management. PS is an essential procedure: clinically, ethically, deontologically and legally. Withholding PS, when clinically indicated, violates the principles of good clinical practice and is ethically, deontologically and legally unjustified.

10.2 The Definition of Palliative Sedation

The European Association of Palliative Care (EAPC) defines 'palliative sedation in the context of palliative medicine as the monitored use of medications intended to induce a state of decreased or absent awareness (unconsciousness) in order to relieve the burden of otherwise intractable suffering in an ethically acceptable way for the patient, family and healthcare providers' [1]. EAPC advice includes directions for the treatment of suffering due to the withdrawal of life-sustaining treatments [1].

Since the publication of the EAPC recommendations, numerous guidelines highlighting differences in the definition of both PS and refractory symptoms have appeared in the literature (2–5).

L. Orsi (✉)
Società Italiana di Cure Palliative, Milan, Italy

Rivista Italiana di Cure Palliative, Milan, Italy
e-mail: orsiluciano@gmail.com

M. Romanò (ed.), *Palliative Care in Cardiac Intensive Care Units*,
https://doi.org/10.1007/978-3-030-80112-0_10

A symptom is defined as refractory when it cannot be adequately controlled through conventional treatment, within an acceptable time span, with a risk-benefit ratio that is acceptable for the patient, with appropriate procedures and support interventions, and without using sedative drugs to reduce consciousness [1–6].

The refractoriness of a symptom is the defining aspect ensuring legitimacy for PS. The care team must therefore acquire and develop the necessary skills; if any doubts regarding a symptom's refractoriness exist, palliative consultation is advised.

The decision to start PS is based on an *imminent death* prognosis that refers to the 'last hours-last days' time span, generally referred to as the last 15 days of life [1, 4].

The incidence of PS in terminal cancer patients ranges between 12% and 16% [7]; less data is available for heart failure patients but it suggests an incidence of up to 40% [8, 9].

10.3 Indications for Palliative Sedation

The main indications for PS in cardiovascular diseases and advanced heart failure (HF) are dyspnoea (19%), terminal delirium (11%), profound general malaise/asthenia (51%), pain (8%) and psycho-existential suffering (8%) [4, 8–11]. Another important indication is the withdrawal of life-sustaining treatments, such as mechanical ventilation, mechanical circulatory support (MCS) and renal replacement therapies (RRT) [1, 8–12].

PS decision-making process and implementation can be problematic, even with clear refractory symptoms, when the care team has poor clinical, communicative/interpersonal and ethical skills. Therefore, all cardiac intensive care unit (CICU) health professionals involved in the management of the terminal phases of advanced heart failure or other chronic diseases should acquire specialised training for this procedure and make use of specialist palliative care consultation.

10.4 Types of Palliative Sedation

Types of PS for the management of refractory symptom suffering are the following:

- **Emergency sedation** [1, 4, 5] is carried out when events that could quickly lead to death have been ascertained and include terminal stages of pulmonary oedema, severe hypoxemic conditions (for example massive pulmonary thromboembolism), irreversible shock and so on. In these cases, the procedure should quickly reduce or remove consciousness via the rapid administration of sedatives at suitable dosages. When death is expected to be close, similar drug administration methods should be carried out while suspending life-sustaining treatments (e.g. the withdrawal of mechanical ventilation).
- **Deep continuous sedation** is the most frequent type of sedation and is performed by progressively increasing sedative dosages as suffering increases. This

is designed to reach a level of sedation that prevents the patient from perceiving any increase in suffering. The concept of proportionality, i.e. the increase in dosage proportional to the intensity of suffering, is fundamental and some authors define this type of sedation 'proportionate palliative sedation' [13–15].

- **Respite or transient sedation** is used when the terminal phases are uncertain or when the refractoriness of a symptom is in doubt or, more frequently, when psycho-existential suffering must be managed in a patient with an estimated prognosis of more than 2 weeks [1, 13–16]. This temporary form of PS is carried out in agreement with the patient (or surrogate decision maker) to reduce consciousness for a short period (for example 12–48 h), with a subsequent gradual reduction in sedative dosage, allowing the patient to regain consciousness and a re-evaluation of the level of suffering.
- **Intermittent sedation** consists of the repetition of respite sedation for recurrent episodes of suffering. If intermittent sedation is unsuccessful, deep continuous sedation must be provided.

Clinical observation of PS is required to ensure appropriate monitoring of the patients' suffering and is implemented using scales such as Richmond Agitation-Sedation Scale (RASS) [17] with clinical observations being repeated over time [1, 2, 14]. The purpose is to monitor the level of suffering rather than to understand the depth of sedation [2, 13, 14].

10.5 Pharmacological Aspects

PS consists of an induction stage where increasing dosages of sedatives are repeatedly administered until suffering is under control, followed by a maintenance stage where dosages are modulated to maintain good overall control of suffering. The provision and administration must include planning for supplementary pharmacological boli (rescue doses) to manage peaks in the intensity of suffering. It is good clinical practice to use a limited number of drugs that are easily manageable, well known to the care team and chosen in line with standard clinical criteria (body weight, age, general conditions, hepatic and renal functions, previous sedative therapy and so on). Specialist advice from a palliative care team may be appropriate in carrying out the first sedations.

The method of administration must avoid any significant use of liquids (to avoid an increase in bronchial secretion, worsening dyspnoea, nausea and vomiting) and, when adjusting sedation dosages to the intensity of suffering, the infusion rate must be taken into account. Hence, in the hospital context, the use of intravenous or subcutaneous syringe pumps is preferable, while the use of diluted medication via intravenous drip is to be avoided due to the risk of introducing excessive quantities of fluids.

Benzodiazepines are the most commonly used sedatives thanks to their anxiolytic, amnesic and anticonvulsant effects, and their sedative synergic action with opiates and antipsychotics. Midazolam is the first-choice sedative in all settings, as reported in literature [1, 2, 5, 14]. Propofol and dexmedetomidine [7, 8] are less used. Generally, maximum sedative dosages are not precisely specified, as PS is designed to achieve and maintain an adequate control over suffering caused by psychophysical symptoms, and can thus be over ten times the normal average dosage [17–19].

In cases where a patient is already being treated with opiates (for example morphine to control dyspnoea or pain) these should not be suspended during PS. In fact, if there is pain or if dyspnoea deteriorates, dosage should be increased.

Table 10.1 Sedative drugs usable in palliative sedation

Medication	Compatibility and warnings	Induction dosage	Maintenance dosage	Route of administration
Benzodiazepine				
Midazolam 1st choice	Opiate, saline solution, dextrose solution	Bolus: 1–5 mg (0.01–0.07 mg/kg) repeatable or 0.5–1 mg/h	10–120 mg/day (0.03–0.1 mg/kg/h) or 1–20 mg/h	Subcutaneous–intravenous
Lorazepam	Opiates, saline solution, dextrose solution	Bolus: 2–4 mg (0.05 mg/kg) repeatable every 2–4 h	0.25–1 mg/h	Subcutaneous–intravenous
Neuroleptics/antipsychotics				
Haloperidol 1st choice	Opiates, midazolam, saline solution	Bolus: 2–5 mg	5–100 mg	Subcutaneous–intravenous
Chlorpromazine		Bolus: 12.5–50 mg or 3–5 mg/h	1–12.5 mg/h 37.5–150 mg/day	Intravenous Intramuscular
Promazine	Opiates, saline solution, dextrose solution	Bolus: 10–50 mg	0.2–2 mg/kg/h (50–70 mg/day)	Intramuscolar Intravenous
General anaesthetics				
Phenobarbital		Bolus: 100–200 mg	10–30 mg/h (600–1200 mg/day)	Subcutaneous–intravenous Intramuscular
Thiopental	Hospital use medication	Bolus: 2–3 mg/kg slowly (<50 mg/min)	1–2 mg/kg/h	Intravenous
Propofol	Hospital use medication	Bolus: 0.5 mg/kg/h (10–50 mg)	0.5–2 mg/kg/h	Intravenous
Dexmedetomidine	4 µg/mL Infusion	Bolus 1 µg/kg in 10 min	0.2–1 µg/kg/h	Intravenous

Modified and published with the permission of the publisher: Orsi [4]

Table 10.1 shows the main drugs and methods of administration used in PS. For further pharmacological information and methods of administration, reference to the specialist literature is recommended [1, 2, 5, 14, 15, 18–20].

10.6 Ethical Aspects in Palliative Sedation

However delicate it may be, sedation in end-of-life palliative care is a 'normal' treatment procedure carried out in the terminal stages of the disease. Indeed, it demands the same ethical and clinical rigor as other treatments [14, 18]. Major ethics theories consider palliative sedation ethically legitimate.

In **principlism ethics**, PS is legitimate when it respects the principle of patient autonomy (self-determination) and where it respects the principles of beneficence (i.e. doing only what is good for the patient) and non-maleficence (i.e. doing no harm to the patient) [21].

In **quality-of-life ethics**, PS is ethically legitimate when it respects patient self-determination and improves the dying process [22].

In **sanctity/inviolability of life ethics**, which forbids interference with the intrinsic finality of human life, PS is justified by the double-effect doctrine and by ethical proportionality criteria [23, 24].

The double-effect doctrine [23, 24] holds that it is entirely moral to carry out treatment that has a beneficial effect (alleviating suffering) and a possible adverse effect (hypothetical shortening of life), provided that the latter is not intentionally sought and there is no alternative treatment. In addition, there should be a proportional relationship between beneficial effect (control of suffering) and adverse effect (hypothetical acceleration of death) insofar as the positive effect must prevail over the negative effect. From this ethical perspective, it is the final stage of the disease and not the sedation that, ultimately, causes the patient's death.

10.7 The Ethical Difference Between Palliative Sedation and Euthanasia

PS is clinically and ethically a radically different treatment procedure to euthanasia [1–5, 14, 22]. Euthanasia is defined as 'a physician (or another person) intentionally killing someone by the administration of drugs, at that person's voluntary and competent request' [1, 25].

PS can clearly be distinguished from euthanasia empirically and ethically by examining three core aspects of the procedure: (1) the treatment aim (intention); (2) types of drugs, dosages and route of administration; and (3) final result.

Regarding the first aspect, it should be noted that the aim (intention) of PS is to control suffering and not to induce the patient's death, in contrast to euthanasia. Regarding the types of drugs, dosages and route of administration used in PS, sedatives or general anaesthetics are employed to proportionately reduce consciousness and not to cause a quick death, as occurs in euthanasia procedures where drugs are used to be lethal. Finally, regarding the third aspect, PS interventions result in patients' reduced perception of suffering, whereas euthanasia leads to the patient's death.

It is worth clarifying that the correct use of sedatives or general anaesthetics, including their use in combination with opiates, does not provoke early death following a serious respiratory depression, as described in comparative studies on sedated and unsedated patients [1, 7, 26, 27].

Despite persistent debate on ethics, it is widely held that palliative sedation differs from euthanasia and is not aimed at accelerating death [27].

10.8 The Relationship Between Palliative Sedation and Forgoing Treatment

Consensual forgoing treatment and PS consist of both withholding new treatments and withdrawing ongoing ones. Although often associated with PS, the decision to forgo treatment is distinct to that of starting PS [1, 5, 19]. Forgoing treatment is motivated by various factors: the proven futility of an ongoing treatment, the ethical non-proportionality of many treatments in terminal stages of illness and the unavailability of oral route of administration for many drugs. The most emotionally problematic ones are those relating to forgoing artificial hydration and nutrition. However, they are fully coherent with PS in the terminal stages of life, because they are no longer clinically advised or even unadvisable due to their pejorative effects on dyspnoea, nausea, vomiting, etc. [1, 14, 18, 28, 29]. In these clinical circumstances, the withdrawal of artificial hydration and nutrition does not determine early death. Cardiovascular diseases and other comorbidities lead to the patient's death [30].

Similar considerations are true for other therapies (infusion of inotropes, vasoactive amines, implantable cardioverter defibrillators, mechanical circulatory supports, mechanical ventilation, renal replacement therapies, extracorporeal membrane oxygenation, anticoagulants, antibiotics and blood transfusion) that become disproportionate or prove futile, or that are knowingly refused by a patient with full decision-making competence [10–12]. The aim of forgoing treatment is to avoid a lengthening of the terminal stages characterised by patient suffering and discomfort. Only those treatments that allow the control of suffering and maximise patient comfort are used in the terminal stages [31].

In short, it can be stated that forgoing all types of treatment is morally legitimate both in terms of quality-of-life ethics (because it improves the well-being of the patient and/or respects autonomy) and in terms of sanctity of life ethics, because it respects the criterion of proportionality [21, 22, 25].

The criterion of proportionality allows the classification of a treatment as increasingly disproportionate, and thus not to be administered. The greater the reduction in the probability of success, the greater the reduction in the quantity or quality of life expectancy and the greater the treatment burden for the patient are the determinants of disproportionality. When treatment is judged disproportionate, it should be neither offered nor carried out since overtreatment is ethically inadmissible. For these fundamental reasons, withholding/withdrawing treatment is not definable as euthanasia [24, 25].

10.9 Correct Decision-Making Management

The ethical-legal criteria to be used with mentally competent patient in the decision-making process is informed consent (IC), whereas shared care planning (SCP), advance directives (AD), substituted judgement and patient best interest are used with mentally incompetent patients. Informed consent is valid with mentally competent patients and is generally continuously sought also beforehand with SCP or AD [32].

In the case of mentally incompetent patients, and in the absence of SCP or AD, the decision to initiate PS is taken by doctors or the substitute decision maker resorting to substituted judgement, based on the patient's wishes previously expressed to family members or care team [33].

If the patient is mentally incompetent and the wishes are unknown or unreconstructible, or in an emergency situation (where it is not possible to obtain IC or AD or formulate a substituted judgement), doctors must resort to the 'best interest' criterion. This criterion is based on the balance between expected benefits and burdens foreseen by the treatment for a specific patient in keeping with the principles of beneficence and non-maleficence. The 'best interest' of a terminally ill patient with refractory symptoms is PS, in that it is good clinical practice [1, 5].

During the decision-making process the caregiver, family members and the patient's emotionally connected entourage should be informed once the patient's permission has been obtained [32, 33].

Significantly, family members' involvement is kept at a strictly informative level. Family members do not have any decision-making power, unless one of the family members is the surrogate decision maker [34].

References

1. Cherny NI, Radbruch L. European Association for Palliative Care (EAPC) recommended framework for the use of sedation in palliative care. Palliat Med. 2009;23(7):581–93.
2. Schildmann E, Schildmann J. Palliative sedation therapy: a systematic literature review and critical appraisal of available guidance on indication and decision making. J Palliat Med. 2014;17:601–11.
3. Raccomandazioni della SICP sulla Sedazione Terminale/Sedazione Palliativa. Rivista Italiana di Cure Palliative 2008;1:16–36. https://www.sicp.it/documenti/sicp/2006/10/raccomandazioni-della-sicp-sulla-sedazione-terminale-sedazione-palliativa/. Accessed June 2020.
4. Orsi L. La sedazione palliativa: definizione, indicazioni, farmaci, aspetti etici e gestionali. In: Romanò M, editor. Scompenso cardiaco e cure palliative. Integrazione e gestione nella pratica clinica quotidiana. Roma: Il Pensiero Scientifico; 2018. p. 253–65.

5. Haute Autoritè de Santé Care Pathway Guide How to implement continuous deep sedation until death? February 2018. https://www.has-sante.fr/upload/docs/application/pdf/2018-11/care_pathway_guide_how_to_implement_continuous_deep_sedation_until_death.pdf. Accessed June 2020.

6. Presidency of the Council of Ministers. National Bioethics Committee. Deep and continuous palliative sedation in the imminence of death; 29 Jan 2016. http://bioetica.governo.it/en/opinions/opinions-responses/deep-and-continuous-palliative-sedation-in-the-imminence-of-death/. Accessed June 2020.

7. Maltoni M, Scarpi E, Nanni O. Palliative sedation for intolerable suffering. Curr Opin Oncol. 2014;26:389–94.

8. Hamatani Y, Nakai E, Nakamura E, Miyata M, Kawano Y, Takada Y, et al. Survey of palliative sedation at end of life in terminally ill heart failure patients—a single-center experience of 5-year follow-up. Circ J. 2019;83(7):1607–11. https://doi.org/10.1253/circj.CJ-19-0125.

9. Kuragaichi T, Kurozumi Y, Ohishi S, Sugano Y, Sakashita A, Kotooka N, et al. Nationwide survey of palliative care for patients with heart failure in Japan. Circ J. 2018;82(5):1336–43. https://doi.org/10.1253/circj.CJ-17-1305. Epub 2018 Mar 10.

10. Romanò M. Facilitating supportive care in cardiac intensive care units. Curr Opin Support Palliat Care. 2020;14(1):19–24.

11. Rady MY, Verheijde JL. Ethical challenges with deactivation of durable mechanical circulatory support at the end of life: left ventricular assist devices and total artificial hearts. J Intensive Care Med. 2014;29(1):3–12. https://doi.org/10.1177/0885066611432415.

12. Wiens EJ, Pilkey J, Wong JK. Delivery of end-of-life care in patients requesting withdrawal of a left ventricular assist device using intranasal opioids and benzodiazepines. J Palliat Care. 2019;34(2):92–5. https://doi.org/10.1177/0825859719829492.

13. Cavanaugh TA. Proportionate palliative sedation and the giving of a deadly drug: the conundrum. Theor Med Bioeth. 2018;39(3):221–31.

14. Royal Dutch Medical Association (KNMG). Guideline for palliative sedation; 2009 https://www.palliativedrugs.com/download/091110_KNMG_Guideline_for_Palliative_sedation_2009__2_%5B1%5D.pdf. Accessed June 2020.

15. Arantzamendi M, Belar A, Payne S, Rijpstra M, Preston N, Menten J, et al. Clinical aspects of palliative sedation in prospective studies. A systematic review. J Pain Symptom Manage. 2020; https://doi.org/10.1016/j.jpainsymman.2020.09.022.

16. Swart SJ, van der Heide A, van Zulen L, Perez RS, Zuurmond WW, van der Maas PJ, et al. Continuous palliative sedation: not only a response to physical suffering. J Pallat Med. 2014;17(1):27–37.

17. Ely EW, Truman B, Shintani A, et al. Monitoring sedation status over time in ICU patients: reliability and validity of the Richmond Agitation-Sedation Scale (RASS). JAMA. 2003;289:2983–91.

18. Morita T, Bito S, Kurihara Y, Uchitomi Y. Development of a clinical guideline for palliative sedation therapy using the Delphi method. J Palliat Med. 2005;8(4):716–29.

19. Claessens P, Menten J, Schotsman P, Broeckaert B. Palliative sedation: a review of the research literature. J Paine Symptom Manage. 2008;36(3):310–33.

20. Hawryluck LA, Harvey RCW, Lemieux-Charles L, Singer PA. Consensus guidelines on analgesia and sedation in dying intensive care unit patients. BMC Med Ethics. 2000;3:3. www.biomedcentral.com/1472-6939/3/3

21. Beauchamp TL, Childress JF. Principles of bioethics. 4th ed. Oxford: Oxford Univ Press; 1994.

22. Engelhardt HT. The foundations of bioethics. 2nd ed. New York: Oxford University Press; 1995.

23. Compendium of the Catechism of the Catholic Church Libreria Editrice Vaticana 2005; § 471. http://www.vatican.va/archive/compendium_ccc/documents/archive_2005_compendium-ccc_en.html

24. The National Catholic Bioethics Center. The new charter for health care workers Online August 2018 © 2018 by The National Catholic Bioethics Center § 149–159, p.122–130.

25. Radbruch L, Leget C, Bahr P, Müller-Busch C, Ellershaw J, de Conno F, et al. Euthanasia and physician-assisted suicide: a white paper from the European Association for Palliative Care.

Palliat Med. 2016;30(2):104–16. https://www.eapcnet.eu/eapc-groups/archives/task-forces-archives/euthanasia/ArtMID/1195/ArticleID/456/euthanasia-and-physician-assisted-suicide-a-white-paper-from-the-european-association-for-palliative-care. Accessed June 2020.

26. Beller EM, van Driel ML, McGregor L, Truong S, Mitchell G. Palliative pharmacological sedation for terminally ill adults. Cochrane Database Syst Rev. 2015;1:CD010206. http://onlinelibrary.wiley.com/doi/10.1002/14651858.CD010206.pub2/abstract;jsessionid=2BAAA489C4FFD85E36CC4991827BC599.f02t03. Accessed June 2020.

27. Sulmasy DP. Sedation and care at the end of life. Theor Med Bioeth. 2018;39:171–80.

28. Kirk TW, Mahon MM. National Hospice and Palliative Care Organization (NHPCO) position statement and commentary on the use of palliative sedation in imminently dying terminally ill patients. J Pain Symptom Manag. 2010;39(5):914–23.

29. Bruera E, Hui D, Dalal S, Torres-Vigil I, Trumble J, Roosth J, et al. Parenteral hydration in patients with advanced cancer: a multicenter, double-blind, placebo-controlled randomised trial. J Clin Oncol. 2013;31(1):111–8.

30. Maeda I, Morita T, Yamaguchi T, Inoue S, Ikenaga M, Matsumoto Y, et al. Effect of continuous deep sedation on survival in patients with advanced cancer (J-Proval): a propensity score-weighted analysis of a prospective cohort study. Lancet Oncol. 2016;17(1):115–22.

31. Downar J, Delaney JW, Hawryluck L, et al. Guidelines for the withdrawal of life-sustaining measures. Intensive Care Med. 2016;42(6):1003–17.

32. Rietjens JAC, Sudore RL, Connolly M, van Delden JJ, Drickamer MA, Droger M, et al. Definition and recommendations for advance care planning: an international consensus supported by the European Association for Palliative Care. Lancet Oncol. 2017;18(9):e543–51.

33. Caulley L, Gillick MR, Lehmann LS. Substitute decision making in end-of-life care. N Engl J Med. 2018;378:2339–41.

34. Sobanski P, Alt-Epping B, Currow D, Goodlin SJ, Grodzicki T, Hogg K, et al. Palliative care for people living with heart failure-European Association for Palliative Care Task Force expert position statement. Cardiovasc Res. 2020;116:12–27.

Nursing and the End of Life in Cardiac Intensive Care Unit (CICU)

11

Rosie Cervera-Jackson and Joanne Tillman

11.1 Introduction

Providing end-of-life care is an important part of the intensive care unit (ICU) nurse's role. Mortality rates in the cardiac intensive care unit (CICU) have been reported at 5.8% [1].

However for specific patient groups, mortality is considerably higher: 40–47% for hospital inpatients with cardiogenic shock [2] and for adult patients receiving extracorporeal cardiopulmonary resuscitation mortality is 41% at discontinuation of extracorporeal life support [3]. The acuity of illness in the CICU patient population has increased over time and, along with it, the proportion of non-cardiovascular comorbidities and multi-organ failure [1]. Nurses are therefore required to facilitate end-of-life care by integrating a palliative care approach into the context of a high-technological environment, primarily designed for the delivery of life-sustaining therapies.

11.2 Decision-Making and Discussions About Goals of Care

Of the patients who die in ICU, over 85% have life-sustaining therapies withheld or withdrawn as part of end-of-life care [4]. The shift in the goals of care occurs after multidisciplinary team (MDT) discussion involving the patient (if conscious) and those close to them. During discussions, caregivers should clearly set out which treatments are futile and what is the likely outcome of continuing them. They must elicit information about the patient's wishes and agree on how and when to

R. Cervera-Jackson (✉) · J. Tillman
Adult Intensive Care Unit, Royal Brompton and Harefield Hospitals, London, UK
e-mail: r.cervera-jackson@rbht.nhs.uk; J.Tillman@rbht.nhs.uk

M. Romanò (ed.), *Palliative Care in Cardiac Intensive Care Units*,
https://doi.org/10.1007/978-3-030-80112-0_11

withdraw or limit life-sustaining therapies and replace them with palliative care interventions. Caregivers should explore with the patient and/or those close to them the existence of advance directives and any nominated power of attorney and, if they exist, they must be consulted as part of the decision-making process. If the patient lacks capacity, and it has not been possible to identify any family or close friends, an independent advocate should be requested to take part in discussions. Referral should be made to the organ donation specialist team to ascertain the potential of the patient to donate organs or tissues after death. If organ donation is a possibility, a member of the organ donation specialist team should be invited to join family discussions, explain the process of deceased organ donation and seek consent. All discussions should include the nursing team as part of the MDT as nurses are well placed to gather relevant information throughout the admission about the patient and their wishes which will form part of end-of-life care discussions.

11.3 Person- and Family-Centred Care

Good end-of-life care is part of patient- and family-centred care. The central role of the nurse in providing end-of-life care was analysed by Sekse et al. [5] in a meta-synthesis which picked out a set of characteristics that made nurses uniquely pivotal in palliative care: *being available, being a coordinator of care for patients and relatives, doing what is needed, being attentively present and dedicated* and *standing in demanding situations.* Nurses provide round-the-clock care at the bedside in CICU and are the professionals who spend the most time with the patient and their families. The therapeutic relationship nurses create with the patient, and those close to them, facilitates good end-of-life care, which meets the patient's physical, psychosocial, emotional and spiritual needs.

It is helpful to obtain and document 'get to know me' information, about the patient's likes, dislikes and what is important to them, during the CICU admission [6].

This is especially important when the patient has been unconscious or unable to communicate during their CICU admission. Encouraging family to bring photographs of the patient and those close to them to place at the bedside is another helpful way of assisting caregivers to see the person beyond the illness, particularly at the end of life. Occasionally, end-of-life care is provided to patients receiving temporary circulatory support who have not experienced cardiac recovery and for whom no destination therapy option exists. These patients are sometimes awake and have the capacity to fully participate in discussions about their care. It is reasonable to offer time to patients in this unusual situation to say goodbye to family and friends and to put their affairs in order while continuing life-sustaining therapy. Interaction with the patient and their family in a way that conserves dignity can be guided by the ABCD mnemonic: attitudes (be aware of how our attitudes and assumptions affect our practice), behaviours (behave respectfully in a manner which honours the importance of patients and their families), compassion (be sensitive to suffering and act to relieve it) and dialogue (encourage dialogue with and between patients and their families) [7].

11.4   Care Planning

When life-sustaining treatment limitation or withdrawal is proposed, it is important to have a clearly documented care plan which is discussed in detail between the medical team and the nurse caring for the patient, as well as any other teams who will be involved, such as supportive and palliative care, electrophysiology (if the patient has a pacemaker or implantable cardioverter defibrillator (ICD), psychology, physiotherapy and spiritual care teams. A 'not for cardiopulmonary resuscitation' order should be created or reviewed for validity. Every treatment should be reviewed and those which are considered to no longer bring benefit to the patient should cease or be limited. The potential for pain and distress at the end of life should be anticipated and provisions made to prevent and treat unpleasant symptoms, thus achieving comfort and dignity. Life-sustaining therapies which might be limited or withdrawn include vasoactive medications, mechanical ventilation, renal replacement therapy, ICD and mechanical circulatory support like venoarterial-extracorporeal membrane oxygenation (ECMO), ventricular assist device, impella or intra aortic balloon pump. A clear plan with timings, roles and responsibilities should be agreed before de-escalation of life-sustaining treatment occurs. Where the dying patient is awake, a shared care plan created together with the CICU team can provide a sense of control and, at the same time, reduces the psychological burden on them [8].

11.5   Palliative Interventions

The primary focus of routine nursing care tasks should shift towards relieving pain and anxiety, and managing respiratory secretions, hunger, thirst and delirium. Providing eye, skin, mouth, hygiene and continence care, pressure area care, and patient positioning should promote comfort and ease respiratory distress. Pain known to be associated with care tasks should be anticipated and pre-emptively treated—for instance, through administration of opioid bolus prior to and after repositioning [9]. Adverse effects of medication should be anticipated and proactively managed. For instance, nausea, pruritis and constipation can occur with opioids but can be managed without limiting pain relief, and should be discussed early with the intensivist, specialist pharmacist and/or palliative care team. Non-pharmacological strategies to reduce pain and anxiety should be considered and include relaxation, massage and music therapies [10].

Regular, repeated assessment and treatment titration are essential. For patients who can self-report, choose the simplest method, such as a numerical or visual analogue scale. For patients who are unable to communicate, use validated assessment tools designed for this purpose. It is important to integrate the results of the assessment into care delivery/planning. For example, signs of distress or agitation could be caused by pain, thirst, respiratory failure or anxiety, or a combination of these. Response to interventions should be closely monitored and can be used to verify the cause of distressing symptoms in situations when assessment is challenging [11, 12]. Increasingly, patients admitted to CICU with acute illness already experience pain, dyspnoea and anxiety as a result of chronic heart failure [13]. Nurses can find out from the patient or those close to them which familiar strategies work at home and try to facilitate them in hospital. A decreasing level of consciousness is normal at the end of life and may be augmented by the requirement for sedatives. Regardless of the patient's level of consciousness, it remains important for caregivers to introduce themselves to the patient, explain what is happening to them and regularly reassure them that they are being looked after and are not alone.

See Table 11.1 for guide to assessment and treatment of symptoms and syndromes experienced by patients at the end of life in CICU.

The time interval between de-escalation or discontinuation of life-sustaining treatment and death is unknowable, so it is important to clearly document assessment and treatment response, to aid handover of care.

11.6 Preparing for Withdrawal of Life-Sustaining Treatment or Imminent Death

The CICU bedside environment can be adapted to meet the needs of the patient and those close to them at the end of life. Removing unneeded technology and devices which may act as barriers between the patient and their family while providing a more private and homely space can enhance the care environment at the end of life [14]. Surplus equipment such as the ventilator or haemofilter can be removed, along with continuous monitoring. Device alarms can be deactivated to promote a calm environment, particularly while mechanical ventilation or temporary circulatory support devices are being withdrawn [13]. Devices must be checked regularly while alarms are off and medication infusion device alarms should remain on. Removal of invasive devices, such as vascular access devices or feeding tubes, can be considered if no longer required and if removing them would not cause pain or distress.

It is preferable for the patient to have a private room, unless moving them would cause pain or distress or hasten their death, where severe cardiovascular or respiratory instability is present. The family can be encouraged to bring in familiar objects from home, such as photographs and blankets [4]. Seating for family should be provided at the bedside and the height of the bed adjusted to it. Lighting should suit the patient and family's preference, music should be offered and the bed can be reoriented—Muslim patients, for instance, might wish to face towards Mecca.

11.7 Meeting Psychosocial and Spiritual Needs

Part of a good death has been described as 'being treated as an individual, with dignity and respect' and 'being in the company of close family and/or friends' [15]. Facilitating the presence of those close to the patient at the end of life is an important aspect of the CICU nurse role, as well as providing support and reassurance

Table 11.1 Bedside assessment tools and interventions for symptoms and syndromes commonly experienced by patients at the end of life in the cardiac intensive care unit

Symptom/ syndrome	Assessment tool for patients who are unable to self-report	Intervention
Pain	Behavioural Pain Scale (BPS) Critical Care Pain Observation Tool (CPOT)	Pharmacological: parenteral opioids titrated to comfort with non-opioid adjuvant, e.g. paracetamol (regularly assess for adverse opioid effects including nausea, pruritis and constipation). Pain, which is refractory to analgesic therapy, might require the addition of sedatives to achieve symptom control (Romanò [13]). Non-pharmacological: relaxation techniques, massage, music therapy
Anxiety/distress/ agitation	Richmond Agitation Sedation Scale (RASS)	First, exclude pain, thirst and adverse effects of medication. Pharmacological: Benzodiazepines Non-pharmacological: relaxation techniques, massage, music therapy, family and/or caregiver presence
Delirium	Confusion Assessment Method-ICU (CAM-ICU)	Pharmacological: antipsychotic medications are not indicated for treatment of critical illness-related delirium Non-pharmacological: multimodal interventions including reorientation, minimising sensory deficits (supplying glasses and hearing aids if usually worn) and family presence
Dyspnoea	Respiratory Distress Observation Scale© (RDOS) (Campbell M 2008)	Pharmacological: provide oxygen therapy for acute hypoxaemia; dyspnoea can be managed with opioids, plus benzodiazepine adjunct if required, and anticholinergics to reduce respiratory secretions, e.g. hyoscine Non-pharmacological: positioning to facilitate easy breathing and expectoration, cool fan
Thirst	Indirect: assess for signs of dehydration, e.g. xerostomia (dry mouth); consider thirst as a potential cause of distress or agitation	Artificial hydration therapy (e.g. IV fluid administration) might be indicated Frequent oral swabs, sterile ice-cold water sprays and application of lip moisturiser should be ensured (Puntillo [12]) Heated humidified oxygen delivery circuit, set at correct temperature for endotracheal/tracheal tube or mask/nasal cannulae (Puntillo [11])
Gastrointestinal discomfort	Assess for signs of nausea or constipation	Pharmacological: anti-emetics (nausea), laxatives (constipation) and/or adjustment of analgesic regime

through giving information about what to expect and what constitutes the normal dying process. Enabling close family and/or friends to take part in care tasks like skin, hair and mouth care, and encouraging them to speak to, hold hands with and share memories with their loved one at the bedside, even if the dying patient is unconscious may provide great comfort. It is often appropriate to relax visiting hours and restrictions on numbers of people at the bedside at the end of life, while monitoring the effect of visiting on the patient. If the patient appears to require rest or quiet time, the nurse should sensitively explain this to the loved ones and readjust visiting recommendations. While a shift from caring for the patient to caring for the family has been noted in the nursing literature, particularly when patients are unconscious, the primary duty of the CICU nurse is to be an advocate to the patient and their needs [4].

As well as providing a private room to the patient at the end of life, and space for family presence, it is also preferable to allocate a separate quiet room nearby for family to gather together, to take turns to spend time at the bedside while providing each other with support away from the bedside. If close family includes children, additional support might be required for their visit, such as a family liaison officer or psychologist. Children and young people, like any family member, should be welcomed to be close to their loved one at the end of life and, with some preparation for the CICU environment, this can be facilitated successfully and positively shape the grieving process [16]. Spiritual support should be explored and if the patient's wishes include a visit by a spiritual representative or a religious ritual before or at the time of death, this should be arranged via the hospital or the family. If families cannot visit, due to distance or travel restrictions, like those experienced during the COVID-19 pandemic, the CICU nurse could consider the option of a virtual visit, for example via videocall. As described by Igra et al. [17], using a set-up like a bedside webcam or designated phone or tablet, with preparation beforehand by a clinical psychologist, enables close family to see their loved one, speak to them and reassure them that they are comfortable and not alone. For patients without visitors, it is the role of the CICU nurse to be present with the patient at the time of death, to ensure that they are accompanied in this final transition with attentiveness and care.

11.8 Unanticipated Death

Unexpected patient deterioration beyond maximal therapy and unanticipated deaths occur in CICU as well as planned withdrawal and limitation of life-sustaining treatment. These fast-moving situations require the nursing team to work together with the rest of the MDT to move from timely treatment escalation and well-coordinated resuscitation to palliation or care after death. It is important to continue to advocate for the patient's wishes; keep the family informed, facilitating their attendance at the bedside where possible; and manage the bedside environment to promote privacy and dignity in death. It is useful to debrief as a team soon after the patient's death (hot debriefing) to enable shared understanding by the healthcare team about what might have precipitated the deterioration [18]. CICU nurses should be invited to take part in the review of the patient's case as part of a scheduled morbidity and mortality review.

11.9   Care After Death

After the patient has died, a doctor should be requested to examine the patient and confirm that death has occurred. The nurse may facilitate a final family visit at the bedside before preparing the patient's body for the mortuary. This involves bathing the patient, closing their eyes and mouth, refitting dentures if available and removing medical devices, if permitted by the coroner/medical examiner. Sternal closure or removal of large devices, like ECMO cannulae, should be arranged with the cardiac surgical or CICU medical team. Clean dressings should be placed over wounds and the body should be dressed in a shroud, wrapped in a sheet and placed into a body bag. The deceased patient's body should be transferred to the mortuary within 4 h of death.

Patient property must be returned to the family, and bereavement information provided. A final interview with the family, attended by the intensivist and the CICU nurse, is recommended to address any concerns or questions about care or the end-of-life process while ensuring that the family's information needs are met. It can be helpful for members of the CICU MDT to also meet to debrief soon after the patient's death, to summarise the patient journey and discuss any concerns or learning points. The senior CICU nurse, such as the shift leader, should meet with the bedside nurse to identify any immediate emotional support needs. While the CICU environment is typically busy and requires all nurses on a shift to be allocated to clinical duties, providing end-of-life care can be distressing; rather than reallocating the nurse to another patient straight away, it might be appropriate to provide some time away from the bedside [19].

CICU nurses who have been involved in end-of-life care may be susceptible to compassion fatigue and moral distress, which are associated with the cumulative losses which may be experienced by healthcare professionals working in acute cardiac care. This susceptibility may be compounded by the unusual situations presented by futility in awake patients on extracorporeal support or unanticipated deterioration and death which also occur in this setting [20]. The consequences of compassion fatigue and moral distress may be worsening mental health and emotional disengagement, which may affect the quality of future care provision [21]. To counteract this, adequate preparation and training prior to providing end-of-life care in CICU, supervision and feedback from a more experienced colleague until sufficient direct experience has been obtained, opportunity to reflect on real and simulated cases and access to psychological assistance are recommended to support CICU nurses in providing end-of-life care.

References

1. Jentzer JC, van Diepen S, Barsness GW, et al. Changes in comorbidities, diagnoses, therapies and outcomes in a contemporary cardiac intensive care unit population. Am Heart J. 2019;215:12–9.
2. van Diepen S, Thiele H. An overview of international cardiogenic shock guidelines and application in clinical practice. Curr Opin Crit Care. 2019;25:365–70.

3. Extracorporeal Life Support Organization. ELSO registry report international summary. Ann Arbor, MI: Extracorporeal Life Support Organization; 2020.
4. Noome M, Genaamd B, Kolmer DM, van Leeuwen E, Dijkstra BM, Vloet LC. The nursing role during end-of-life care in the intensive care unit related to the interaction between patient, family and professional: an integrative review. Scand J Caring Sci. 2016;30(4):645–61.
5. Sekse RJT, Hunskår I, Ellingsen S. The nurse's role in palliative care: a qualitative meta-synthesis. Clin Nurs. 2018;27:e21–38.
6. http://depts.washington.edu/eolcare/products/communication-tools/.
7. Cook D, Rocker G. Dying with dignity in the intensive care unit. N Engl J Med. 2014;370:2506–14.
8. Sprung CL, Truog RD, Curtis, et al. Seeking worldwide professional consensus on the principles of end-of-life care for the critically ill. The Consensus for Worldwide End-of-Life Practice for Patients in Intensive Care Units (WELPICUS) study. Am J Respir Crit Care Med. 2014;190:855–66.
9. Robleda G, Roche-Campo F, Sendra MÀ, et al. Fentanyl as pre-emptive treatment of pain associated with turning mechanically ventilated patients: a randomized controlled feasibility study. Intensive Care Med. 2016;42:183–91.
10. Devlin JW, Skrobik Y, Gélinas C, et al. Clinical practice guidelines for the prevention and management of pain, agitation/sedation, delirium, immobility, and sleep disruption in adult patients in the ICU. Crit Care Med. 2018;46:e825–73.
11. Puntillo K, Nelson JE, Weissman D, et al. Palliative care in the ICU: relief of pain, dyspnea, and thirst. Report from the IPAL-ICU Advisory Board. Intensive Care Med. 2014;40:235–48.
12. Puntillo K, Arai SR, Cooper B, et al. A randomized clinical trial of an intervention to relieve thirst and dry mouth in intensive care unit patients. Intensive Care Med. 2014;40:1295–302.
13. Romanò M. The role of palliative care in the cardiac intensive care unit. Healthcare. 2019;7:30.
14. Efstathiou N, Walker W. Intensive care nurses' experiences of providing end-of-life care after treatment withdrawal: a qualitative study. J Clin Nurs. 2014;23:3188–96.
15. Department of Health. End of life care strategy: promoting high quality care for adults at the end of their life; July 2008.
16. Hanley JR, Piazza J. A visit to the intensive care unit: a family-centered culture change to facilitate pediatric visitation in an adult intensive care unit. Crit Care Nurs Q. 2012;35:113–22.
17. Igra A, McGuire H, Naldrett I, et al. Rapid deployment of virtual ICU support during the COVID-19 pandemic. Future Healthc J. 2020;7:181–4.
18. Clark R, McLean C. The professional and personal debriefing needs of ward based nurses after involvement in a cardiac arrest: an explorative qualitative pilot study. Intensive Crit Care Nurs. 2018;47:78–84.
19. Kisorio LC, Langley GC. End-of-life care in intensive care unit: Family experiences. Intensive Crit Care Nurs. 2016;35:57–6.
20. Pattison N, Marsden R. The morality of good end-of-life care in critical care. Nurs Crit Care. 2017;22:123–4.
21. Walker W, Efstathiou N. Support after patient death in the intensive care unit: Why 'I' is an important letter in grief. Nurs Crit Care. 2020;25:266–8.

Conflict Management in the Cardiac Intensive Care Unit

12

Kateřina Rusinová and Jan Bělohlávek

12.1 Conflicts in the Cardiac Intensive Care Unit: Definitions, Background, and Examples

Conflicts and disagreements are normal part of human communication in stressful situations. Current understanding of conflicts labels them having both negative and positive impacts. The question of conflict is primarily addressed and largely explored by social sciences, mainly psychology. The term "conflict" in a psychological background is usually defined as a process that begins when one party perceives its interests, norms, and values or opinions and viewpoints being opposed, hurt, or encountered by another [1].

There are three groups of general themes that can be found usually underneath a conflict or disagreement in any relationship [2]:

1. Power and control
2. Closeness and care
3. Respect and recognition

The area of healthcare, especially the intensive care unit (ICU), is susceptible to conflict emergence and escalation due to highly complex medical decisions in life-threatening conditions and often highly emotionally loaded patients' life stories. In

K. Rusinová (✉)
Department of Palliative Medicine, First Faculty of Medicine, Charles University, General University Hospital, Prague, Czech Republic
e-mail: katerina.rusinova@lf1.cuni.cz

J. Bělohlávek
Department of Cardiology, First Faculty of Medicine, Charles University, General University Hospital, Prague, Czech Republic
e-mail: Jan.Belohlavek@vfn.cz

M. Romanò (ed.), *Palliative Care in Cardiac Intensive Care Units*,
https://doi.org/10.1007/978-3-030-80112-0_12

a cardiac intensive care unit (CICU), common types of conflict arise on several levels, i.e., inter-teams, intra-team, and with the patients and patients' relatives.

Here let us cite some examples specific for the CICU to illustrate the themes mentioned above. The care of cardiac patients often involves more teams—not only cardiologists: general ICU specialists, anesthesiologists, etc. Each of them comes with a different set of experiences and expectations, but also cognitive biases potentially contributing to a conflict or disagreement [3].

Example 1: Extensive percutaneous coronary or structural intervention followed by a complicated course leads to disagreement on further extent/intensity of therapy. Interventionalists who invested effort and devices may often tend to insist on continued care. An endowment effect might be used as a parallel to explain this phenomenon. It refers to the following: if we feel a sense of psychological *"ownership of the performed intervention"* we may be willing to *"spend more"* on it. In contrast the intensivists coming to the situation "with new eyes" suggest often substantially limited care approach. This could mirror another interesting phenomenon called confirmation bias—they see the sickest patients with worst outcomes significantly more often; hence they may tend to seek information and evidence that support their existing beliefs.

Example 2: Specialists outside the cardiac intensive care express exceedingly high expectations when cardiac complication evolves (acute heart failure/myocardial infarction/cardiac arrest in other chronic disease scenarios) leading to disappointment on further extent of therapy. Cardiologists may experience in these situations what is called *authority bias*. Authority bias is the tendency to attribute greater accuracy to the opinion of an authority figure (unrelated to its content).

Example 3: The rapid dynamics of care intensity changes is another characteristic aspect of the CICU. Care delivery swings between extensive and limited approach, with changing of approaches within short periods of time. During the day, morning rounds may limit the care and later intensivist on call increases the dose of vasopressors despite the agreed-upon treatment plan. Incomplete takeover of care plan is a typical source of conflicts.

Example 4: Different opinions, attitudes, and wording of nursing staff vs. physicians potentially bring friction if not debriefed routinely and timely. The COVID era of intensive care frankly proved the necessity of a high-quality communication with the relatives of critically ill patients. Challenge to achieve trustworthy relationships due to the lack of personal contact in the context of restricted patient visits yields room for misunderstandings, unrealistic expectations, and potential conflicts.

12.2 Conflict Characteristics

Most of the conflicts occur either between families and ICU staff members [4] or within the ICU team [5]. Intra-family conflicts or conflicts with patients are less frequent. When the ICU stay is prolonged, nearly one-third (31.8%) of patients experience conflict associated with their care as shown by a study by Studdert et al. [6] where nurses detected all types of conflict more frequently than physicians, especially intra-team conflicts.

In complicated acute coronary syndromes or cardiac arrest, it is a communicational challenge and a skill how to explain the reality of being "completely" healthy and within minutes to hours in a life-threatening condition so that relatives can understand. Their initial denial—a physiological coping mechanism—might be interpreted by a physician as "they are not willing to understand despite my repeated explanations." This often leads to distrust—a major barrier in honest communication often followed by conflict about goals of care.

Many sources of conflict have been identified in intensive care units. In the Conflicus study [7], half of the intra-team conflicts were related to the end-of-life issues. Poor communication (in quality and in quantity) [8] and general and interpersonal behavior are the most frequent and critical problems creating conflicts. The family, in terms of communication in the context of shifting from curative to palliative care, needs timely information, honesty, and need for clinicians to be clear and to listen [9]. When these needs are unmet, they frequently contribute to a conflict emergence and may facilitate nurses' frustration toward physicians' authority [10]. Every disagreement about the goals of care was found as a major source of conflict in a study by Danjoux Meth et al. [10].

12.3 Managing Conflicts: Can We Be Better In Conflicts?

The question of utmost importance is not merely the conflict itself, which is "a must," even obligatory, but the "repair" [11]. How can we minimize some of the negative escalations? Like in a lot of conflicts outside of healthcare context, we can observe a cyclic "toxic" pattern:

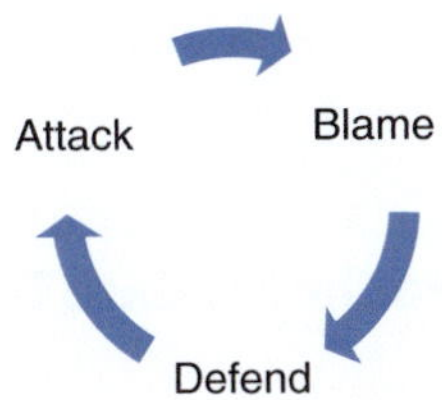

Let us take again an example: a patient in cardiogenic shock on extensive pharmacological support with uncertain neurological status evolves into hemodynamic instability: decision to proceed with mechanical support may be influenced by many related circumstances and cognitive biases: the physician on call might not be trained in mechanical support implantation, or might have a different attitude to the patient's condition or might be reluctant to undertake negative decision (no implant) in a patient that was considered to be perspective for full curative therapy.

To prevent later conflicts, such a decision should be team derived and discussed despite logistical challenges during the process (emergence, unavailability of the specialist, nighttime, etc.). Therefore, several initiatives have been suggested and are becoming widely adopted not only to improve patient outcomes, but also to overcome potential intra-team conflicts [12, 13].

Detailed concept of conflict function, role, and management is derived from non-intensive care literature [1] and is poorly studied in ICU setting [14–16]. Further qualitative and interdisciplinary research is needed to better understand the typology of ICU-specific conflicts, classification of their severity, and impact in terms of both usefulness and harmfulness [17].

Recently, a promising simulation experiment method was introduced to evaluate and study important communication skills of ICU clinicians [18]. Using best practice guidelines and an iterative, multidisciplinary approach, a simulation involving a critically ill patient was developed and refined. This model, shown to be feasible, acceptable, and realistic, opens an opportunity to an in-depth understanding of conflict in ICUs.

Conflict creates a kind of "contraction or stiffness." From a psychological point of view, there is no flexibility, no nuance, no "possible," just "categorical." A lot of what is presented as a fact is rather an intensification of someone's experience. And often, other psychological mechanisms play a role: behind many angers, there is often a hurt involved, as well as behind many criticisms an unspoken wish can be found [19].

So far, only limited number of studies have tested interventions aimed at conflict reduction specifically. Burns et al. evaluated the intervention of social workers in the ICU, who intervened as facilitators of family-ICU staff communication and gave feedback to the clinical team [20]. This intervention, however, failed to demonstrate an effect on satisfaction of care, information, or involvement in the decision-making process.

Although there is yet not any known effective intervention reducing ICU conflicts based on clinical research, the field of ICU communication is well studied and evidence-based recommendations are available about structured communication and family conferences [21].

12.4 Involvement of a Palliative Care Team: Experiences

Palliative care team involvement in daily routine of CICU is becoming a must in comprehensive curative and supportive care [22].

Patient spectrum in high-dependency CICUs changed considerably during the last years and more patients with narrowed or even exhausted therapeutic options are admitted (terminal heart failure, extracorporeal cardiopulmonary resuscitation scenarios, destination pharmacological or mechanical support without exit strategy, etc.). This fact brings new challenges for healthcare professionals and often requires integrating palliative care with social, communicational, ethical, spiritual, and logistical skills and expertise.

Palliative care team should be involved timely to prevent later divergencies and conflicts both within the CICU team and in relation to family or relatives. Patient's and family values and preferences should be discussed early and communicated among the cardiac and palliative care teams to achieve a greater benefit for patients in terms of quality of life, anxiety, depression, and spiritual well-being [23]. Cardiac teams are occasionally reluctant to involve palliative care team being perceived as a therapeutical failure. This is one of the well-described barriers to palliative care [24].

Prevailingly technical understanding of the patient "*therapeutical journey*" must be carefully and repeatedly communicated with interventionalists to prevent mechanistical binary interpretation of actual condition and concurrent processes. Reducing complex problems to their technical aspect might be an example of a lost opportunity to aim, consider, discuss, and apply those therapeutical options that fit well to the patient "*life journey*" [25].

Similarly, this kind of barriers to implement early palliative care also include the patient herself/himself and her/his understanding of the disease trajectory ("*I came for valve change, not to discuss my social, emotional, or spiritual values …*") and the family ("*His family physician recommended coronary angiography and revascularization, did you perform, what was requested? Why are you talking to us about our view of my father´s living will?*").

12.5 How to Turn Conflict into an Opportunity for Improvement?

In other words, we could ask: How could we turn it around so that people can actually hear each other? How to increase our ability for active listening, being aware of our and others' cognitive biases to better manage conflicts? One of the options for conflict resolution is the process of negotiation. Therefore, the skill of interpersonal communication is one of the most important individual qualities. Conscious approach to techniques of negotiations includes several well-described strategies [26]: stay in control under pressure, defuse anger and hostility, listen, explore and understand what the other side really wants, reach agreements that satisfy both sides' needs (win-win scenarios), etc.

For example, discussing treatment plan in case of unfavorable prognosis or end of life is a situation known to be associated with increased risk of conflict emergence [7] and hence requires a careful negotiation. It has been demonstrated that not only knowledge (about advance directive laws, training on how to deliver bad news, etc.) but also what can be called perceived self-efficacy in discussions plays a major role in the ability to attend to the emotional needs of patients and surrogates and succeed in this negotiation process [27]. This finding, so far unidentified by available qualitative research in the field of ICU conflicts, clearly illustrates how complex it is to get a deeper insight into the problem of negotiation in the context of critical illness and highlights the importance of multimodal research design in this area.

12.6 Conclusion

Management of conflicts relies mainly on the principles of social sciences and has not yet been sufficiently explored in CICU; so far only limited number of educational interventions aimed at improving CICU intensivists' ability to handle conflicts have been tested.

The problem of conflicts in the CICU is a complex issue involving specific social skills and requiring knowledge and practice of specific communication strategies. This suggests that while better insight through continuing high-quality research is necessary, it will be crucial to develop targeted medical education to improve conflict management.

References

1. de DCKW, Gelfand MJ, editors. The psychology of conflict and conflict management in organizations. New York; London: Lawrence Erlbaum Associates; 2008. p. 484.
2. Perel E. What couples therapy can teach us about conflict in the workplace. Available online: https://estherperel.com/blog/conflict-in-the-workplace. Accessed 5 April 2021.
3. Saposnik G, Redelmeier D, Ruff CC, et al. Cognitive biases associated with medical decisions: a systematic review. BMC Med Inform Decis Mak. 2016;16(1):138.
4. Abbott KH, Sago JG, Breen CM, et al. Families looking back: one year after discussion of withdrawal or withholding of life-sustaining support. Crit Care Med. 2001;29(1):197–201.
5. Ferrand E, Lemaire F, Regnier B, et al. Discrepancies between perceptions by physicians and nursing staff of intensive care unit end-of-life decisions. Am J Respir Crit Care Med. 2003;167(10):1310–5.
6. Studdert DM, Mello MM, Burns JP, et al. Conflict in the care of patients with prolonged stay in the ICU: types, sources, and predictors. Intensive Care Med. 2003;29(9):1489–97.
7. Azoulay E, Timsit J-F, Sprung CL, et al. Prevalence and factors of intensive care unit conflicts: the Conflicus study. Am J Respir Crit Care Med. 2009;180(9):853–60.
8. Rusinova K, Kukal J, Simek J, et al. Limited family members/staff communication in intensive care units in the Czech and Slovak Republics considerably increases anxiety in patients' relatives—the DEPRESS study. BMC Psychiatry. 2014;14:21.
9. Norton SA, Tilden VP, Tolle SW, et al. Life support withdrawal: communication and conflict. Am J Crit Care Off Publ Am Assoc Crit-Care Nurses. 2003;12(6):548–55.
10. Danjoux Meth N, Lawless B, Hawryluck L. Conflicts in the ICU: perspectives of administrators and clinicians. Intensive Care Med. 2009;35(12):2068–77.
11. NHS. Conflict resolution. Available online: https://www.newarkandsherwoodccg.nhs.uk/media/26793/conflict-resolution-level-1-workbook.pdf. Accessed 5 April 2021.
12. Basir MB, Schreiber T, Dixon S, et al. Feasibility of early mechanical circulatory support in acute myocardial infarction complicated by cardiogenic shock: the Detroit cardiogenic shock initiative. Catheter Cardiovasc Interv. 2018;91(3):454–61.
13. Baran DA, Grines CL, Bailey S, et al. SCAI clinical expert consensus statement on the classification of cardiogenic shock: this document was endorsed by the American College of Cardiology (ACC), the American Heart Association (AHA), the Society of Critical Care

Medicine (SCCM), and the Society of Thoracic Surgeons (STS) in April 2019. Catheter Cardiovasc Interv. 2019;94(1):29–37.

14. Strack van Schijndel RJM, Burchardi H. Bench-to-bedside review: leadership and conflict management in the intensive care unit. Crit Care Lond Engl. 2007;11(6):234.

15. Hawryluck LA, Espin SL, Garwood KC, et al. Pulling together and pushing apart: tides of tension in the ICU team. Acad Med J Assoc Am Med Coll. 2002;77(10 Suppl):S73–6.

16. Lingard L, Espin S, Evans C, et al. The rules of the game: interprofessional collaboration on the intensive care unit team. Crit Care Lond Engl. 2004;8(6):R403–8.

17. Fassier T, Azoulay E. Conflicts and communication gaps in the intensive care unit. Curr Opin Crit Care. 2010;16(6):654–65.

18. Chiarchiaro J, Schuster RA, Ernecoff NC, et al. Developing a simulation to study conflict in ICUs. Ann Am Thorac Soc. 2015;12(4):526–32.

19. Lenski T. Behind every criticism is a wish. Available online: https://tammylenski.com/behind-every-criticism-is-a-wish/. Accessed 5 April 2021.

20. Burns JP, Mello MM, Studdert DM, et al. Results of a clinical trial on care improvement for the critically ill. Crit Care Med. 2003;31(8):2107–17.

21. Curtis JR, White DB. Practical guidance for evidence-based ICU family conferences. Chest. 2008;134(4):835–43.

22. Romano' M. The role of palliative care in the cardiac intensive care unit. Healthcare (Basel). 2019;7(1):30.

23. Rogers JG, Patel CB, Mentz RJ, et al. Palliative care in heart failure: The PAL-HF randomized, controlled clinical trial. J Am Coll Cardiol. 2017;70(3):331–41.

24. Bennardi M, Diviani N, Gamondi C, et al. Palliative care utilization in oncology and hemato-oncology: a systematic review of cognitive barriers and facilitators from the perspective of healthcare professionals, adult patients, and their families. BMC Palliat Care. 2020;19(1):47.

25. Heifetz R, Linsky M. A survival guide for leaders. Harvard Business Review. Available online: https://hbr.org/2002/06/a-survival-guide-for-leaders. Accessed 5 April 2021.

26. Ury W. Getting past no: negotiating with difficult people. Bantam Books: New York; 1991. p. 161.

27. Sulmasy DP, Sood JR, Ury WA. Physicians' confidence in discussing do not resuscitate orders with patients and surrogates. J Med Ethics. 2008;34(2):96–101.

Ethical Considerations in the Use of Technology in the Cardiac Intensive Care Unit

13

Bjørn Hofmann

13.1 Introduction

The tremendous technological progress in medicine in general, and in cardiology in particular, has substantially extended medicine's ability to help people. A broad range of innovations have increased the odds of surviving very critical conditions. However, at the same time as technology has widely extended the possibility of doing good, it also expands the risk of doing harm [1]. Despite Mae West's alleged claim [2], too much of a good thing is not wonderful [3]. At the same time as technology is a fantastic means to extend lives it can extend suffering. The same aggressive and expensive treatments that can do good can come to prolong pain and delay inevitable death.

Due to its fabulous achievements the possibilities of technology have become evermore worshiped, but also hyped and overrated. In technology and progress, we trust. However, in order to apply technology in an appropriate way—helping and not harming people—we need to reflect on the power, goals, and implications of technology—especially when handling the physiologically vital and historically most venerated organ of human beings: the heart.

In this chapter, I will discuss the distinction between utility and futility of medical technology as well as the question of when to start and when to stop treatment (i.e., withholding versus withdrawing). These issues go to the ethical core of medicine: doing good and avoiding harm. Given the extensive potential of modern technology, there are ample chances of futile diagnostics and treatment, and thereby

B. Hofmann (✉)
Department of Health Sciences, Faculty of Medicine and Health Sciences,
Norwegian University of Science and Technology, Gjøvik, Norway

Centre for Medical Ethics, Institute of Health and Society, Faculty of Medicine,
University of Oslo, Oslo, Norway
e-mail: bjoern.hofmann@ntnu.no

M. Romanò (ed.), *Palliative Care in Cardiac Intensive Care Units*,
https://doi.org/10.1007/978-3-030-80112-0_13

prospects to violate the principles of beneficence, non-maleficence, and justice. The great potential of technology also spurs extensive hype, hope, and hubris. In order to bar inappropriate technology use in cardiac intensive care units (as in health care in general) we need to identify and address the drivers of excessive technology use. In this chapter I will address "external" and "internal" drivers in terms of stakeholders and their roles, as well as biases and imperatives as they can undermine autonomy for patients, professionals, and policy makers.

13.2 Utility Versus Futility

Historically very many of the most heated ethical debates in modern medicine stem from the ICU setting. The rapidly expanding possibilities to compensate for biological function failure made it possible to save lives and help people in unprecedented ways. Respirators, defibrillators, dialysis machines, and monitoring devices are but a few examples. The beneficence of technology in the ICU was magnificent. However, at the same time these fantastic possibilities also raised the question of when to stop. What is enough? When do we go from reducing suffering to extending it? When is it appropriate to let people die? What is enough treatment?

Karen Ann Quinlan was one of the first cases that gained attention in the international literature [4]. An interesting debate on futility in medicine [4–14] and in the ICU followed [4, 11, 15–20]. Setting the limits between utility and futility has never been easy and many definitions have been provided in order to clarify the distinction. A Policy Statement from the Society of Critical Care Medicine Ethics Committee defines futile and potentially inappropriate treatments in the following way: "ICU interventions should generally be considered inappropriate when there is no reasonable expectation that the patient will improve sufficiently to survive outside the acute care setting, or when there is no reasonable expectation that the patient's neurologic function will improve sufficiently to allow the patient to perceive the benefits of treatment" [21].

In explicating futility, a useful distinction has been made between quantitative and qualitative futility. *Quantitative futility* is where the likelihood that an intervention will benefit the patient is exceedingly poor, and *qualitative futility* is where the quality of benefit an intervention will produce is exceedingly poor [5, 22]. Hence, one type of futility stems from the fact that the chances of obtaining a goal are small, and another from the fact that the value of obtaining the goals is small. Thus, even if we obtain a goal, the benefit may be negligible or negative [7].

Therefore, the futility debate goes to the ethical core of medicine: doing good and avoid doing harm. Futile treatment violates the principle of beneficence and non-maleficence [23]. Additionally, it may undermine the principle of justice, as ICU treatment is resource demanding and draws resources from other patients [19, 24].

13.3   When to Start and When to Stop: Withholding Versus Withdrawing

The (f)utility issue is practically experienced in the daily clinical question of when to start and when to stop treatment. The vast possibilities of diagnostics and treatment come together with diagnostic and prognostic uncertainty [25] to pose a wide range of ethical dilemmas [26] also discussed in Chaps. 7–11. Moreover, once a treatment has started, it can be difficult to stop.

In the field of cardiac intensive care this is clearly seen in the deactivation of implanted cardioverter-defibrillator devices [27, 28]. These are fantastic devices that may save lives, but also prolong pain and suffering. For reasons to be discussed below it appears easier to start the treatment (implantation and activation) than to stop (deactivation). However, the example illustrates how important the beginnings are—both with respect to using technologies in the individual case and when implementing technologies in general [29]. Every appropriate start of using technology includes a reflection on when to maintain and when to stop.

Both withholding and withdrawing life-preserving treatment are ethically challenging as the consequences are fatal. However, there is an experienced, ethical [30], and epistemic [31] difference between withholding and withdrawing. Besides, withholding or withdrawing life-preserving treatment does not mean "no treatment." The alternative to aggressive treatment is high-quality palliative treatment [32, 33].

13.4   Hype, Hope, and Hubris

The fantastic possibilities provided by modern technology have spurred great optimism with respect to what medicine can do. This comes together with difficulties of discerning utility from futility and a wide range of drivers of technology use to be discussed below. The result is what has been coined "too much medicine" [34–43]. The means of medicine are used beyond their benefit.

Against this, a wide range of measures have been launched to harness medical overactivity and obstruct the overuse of technology. Slow Medicine (IT), Choosing Wisely (global), NICE's "DoNotDo" Database (UK), Preventing Overdiagnosis (UK, USA, then global), Right Care Movement (Lown Institute, USA), Smarter Medicine (CH), Prudent Health Care (Wales, UK), and Wiser Healthcare (AUS) are but a few examples [44, 45].

Despite these timely and impressive efforts, there seems to be a massive overuse of technology that is difficult to control [46–51]. Hubris comes together with hope and generates spin and hype. In order to address these issues, we have to understand the driving forces behind the "too much medicine" phenomenon, and in particular the problem of "too much technology" [52].

13.5 The External Drivers of Too Much Technology

There are many ways of classifying the drivers of technology in health care [53–55]. One way is by analyzing the agents and actors involved in technology use in health care. Clearly *professionals* are involved. Technology has significantly expanded the power of professionals (both for good and bad, as pointed out above). Moreover, professionals have (together with society) extended the field of their subject matter. By addressing evermore ordinary life experiences, medicine has come to medicalize a wide range of phenomena [56]. Additionally, technology plays a key role in what has been called defensive medicine. Even more, professional identity is related to the ability to act which also spurs technology use.

Another technology-driving force is the expansion of the *concept of disease* [57]. Technology has played a decisive role in the expansion of disease definitions ("disease creep") and in including (unpredictable) early stages in disease definitions. Moreover, various types of specialties have been branding of "their" disease entities.

Industry clearly is a driving force in the use as well as in the misuse of technology in health care. The latter happens when improving and promoting tests and treatments beyond benefit, but also when focusing on surrogate outcomes [58] instead of what matters to people. Moreover, disease mongering is well described in the literature [59, 60].

Patients certainly are a driving force in the use of technology in health care. As patients, we are more informed, request more, are more worried, and are more focused on health than ever before. Technology has a high standing and is associated with quality, and we therefore demand advanced tests and treatments. The "popularity paradox" makes us thankful for being "saved" even when technology has overdiagnosed, overtreated, and harmed us, for example when we think that we have been saved from dying from cancer when we have actually been overdiagnosed and overtreated [61].

Feedback loops also reinforce the use of technology. Together with health professionals, industry can develop ever-better diagnostics. However, more accurate tests may find more cases, including more milder cases of disease. When subsequently treating more milder cases of a specific disease, the success rate increases. Increased success makes us invest more in diagnostics and treatment [52], and the loop continues.

Media also is a driving force in technology use in health care. Media often focuses on unjust care, but also on conflicts and polarizations. What is dramatic is exposed more than the chronic. Too little medicine or ignored cases get more attention than exaggerated treatment and care. Not treating a patient with a cardiac condition that could have been treated gains more attention than futile treatment.

Correspondingly, law plays a role in technology use. Law drives the need for documentation, and thus diagnostic testing (and sometimes treatment). Fear of litigation drives defensive medicine and extensive technology use [62, 63].

Figure 13.1 provides a summary of the various drivers of inappropriate technology use.

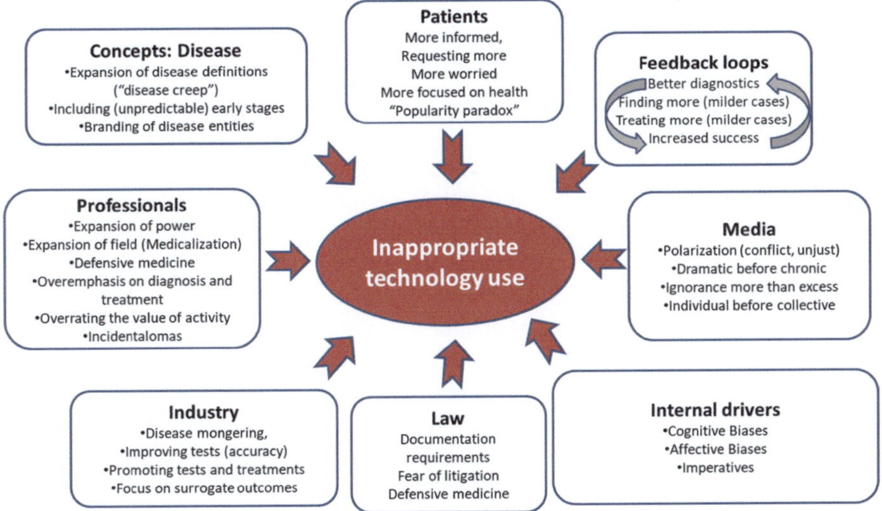

Fig. 13.1 Drivers of inappropriate technology use

13.6 The Internal Drivers of Too Much Technology

In addition to drivers related to stakeholders and actors (and their roles), there are also many drivers internal to these stakeholders and actors. That is, as human beings we have cognitive and affective biases as well as imperatives that drive the implementation and use of technologies in health care. As pointed out by Kahneman and Twersky [64–66], System 1 thinking can be useful when we need to respond and act quickly, but can trick us and lead our decisions astray. In the following, I will highlight some such effects relevant for our (inappropriate) use of technology based on previous studies [67–70].

When we have implemented and have integrated the use of a given technology in practical use, it is hard to stop using it (decommissioning, disinvestment, end using). This effect can be related to cognitive biases such as status quo bias, aversion to change, loss aversion, and endowment effect. Due to these mechanisms, we need to make proper assessments before and under implementing technologies.

Related to this, we tend to have an "adoption addiction" to technology [71]. That is, we seem to be more prone to adoption than to rejection of technologies, more positive to assessment than to reassessment and de-adoption [72]. This relates to the hype and hope effects described above.

Biases, such as aversion to risk, aversion to ambiguity, and anticipated decision regret [73], may make us use technology to "better be safe than sorry." Of course, if this betters the benefits to the patient, that is great. However, if it does not—or makes us to treat our own uncertainty more than the patients' disease—we go astray.

Another effect that may distort rational technology use in health care is fear aversion asymmetry. We tend to be more afraid of doing too little than doing too much—of underdoing than overdoing. This relates to "the popularity paradox" discussed above.

While the biases mentioned so far are mainly cognitive biases (and it can be difficult to differentiate between cognitive and affective biases), affective biases can also influence technology use. One such bias may be called professional identity bias and comes from the fact that professional identity is constituted by action and not by inaction.

This connects to what has been called progress bias [70], as progress is conceived of as a good thing (value) in itself. We tend to have a drive for novelty, and our gut feeling tells us that "new is better than old." Of course, the new technology oftentimes is better than the old, but that is because of its effectiveness and not because of its novelty. These effects relate to the more general trend of technology optimism [70] and can (together with hubris and hope) promote hype and overuse.

Technology optimism is one reason why we connect status and prestige to technologies and to diseases and specialties where we use technologies [74, 75]. Diseases of the heart have high professional prestige [75] and the CICU definitely is a place of high-end use of technology. Using technology because of its high status and prestige, and not because of its benefit to patients, can definitely be unethical.

Imperatives are a third type of human inclination (which resides between System 1 and System 2) [76, 77]. One prominent imperative in the handling of medical technology is the imperative of action according to which action is better (and more integrity promoting) than inaction. This relates to professional identity bias (discussed above) but also to the Latin saying *ut aliquid fiat* ("for something to happen") previously widely taught at medical schools. It also relates to the imperative of possibility, i.e., "can do will do." We have to implement and use a technology, because it is possible.

On an anecdotal note, I was working in a hospital in the 1990s where it became urgent to implement Swan-Ganz monitoring on most patients. The studies documenting the advantage of this were few and of poor quality. Nonetheless, it was imperative to implement the technology. After a while the technology became obsolete. When I asked why they stopped using it, I got no good answer, but apparently new and better technologies had emerged [78].

According to the imperative of complexity "advanced approaches are better than simple" and according to the imperative of extension, "more is better than little." Again, extensive and complex technologies can be better than small and simple ones, but not because of their extension and complexity.

The imperative of knowledge (as well as the fear of uncertainty) may make us take more tests than necessary and treat more than beneficial, and the boys-and-toys effect may make us implement technologies because they are cool [70].

Table 13.1 provides a summary of the various types of cognitive and affective biases and imperatives that undermine appropriate technology use. The point is not that these mechanisms are always bad. They certainly can help us in everyday decision-making. However, these mechanisms can also lead us astray making decisions with technology implementation and use that are not beneficial to patients and even harmful. Moreover, they can undermine autonomy both for patients, professionals, and policy makers. Patient autonomy are not aware of the limitations of the technologies and professionals and policy makers may be mislead by biases and imperatives.

Table 13.1 Overview of various mechanisms undermining appropriate technology implementation and use. The table is based on a submitted paper with the title Internal barriers to efficiency: why disinvestments are so difficult. Identifying and addressing internal barriers to disinvestment of health technologies

Type of mechanism	Mechanism (bias/ imperative)	Short description
Cognitive biases	Status quo bias/aversion to change	"What we have is better than what we will get."
	Risk perception bias	Underestimating risk and overestimating benefits
	Anchoring effect	What you have sets the standard/reference
	Framing effect	We decide on options based on the way they are presented (e.g., with positive or negative connotations)
	The endowment effect	Overvaluing what we have, tendency to retain an object
	Loss aversion effect	Disliking to reduce or lose things or services
	Aversion to risk and aversion to ambiguity	Disliking risk and/or uncertainty
	Better safe than sorry, anticipated decision regret, fear aversion asymmetry	Acting out of fear for the consequences of not doing anything Fear of doing too little > fear of doing too much
Affective biases	Professional identity bias	Professional identity is connected to action and not to inaction
	Progress bias	Progress is a good thing (value) in itself. "New is better than old"
	Status and prestige of diseases, specialties, and technologies	Preferring diseases, services, or technologies due to their status or prestige
Imperatives	Imperative of action, imperative of possibility, Roemer's law	Action is better (and more integrity promoting) than inaction (*ut uliquiad fiat*). Because something *is* possible, it should be implemented. "A built bed is a filled bed"
	Imperative of complexity	"Advanced is better than simple"
	Imperative of extension	"More is better than little"
	Positive feedback loops	Technology use is self-reinforcing
	Imperative of knowledge	Knowledge (testing) is better than ignorance
	White elephants	Technologies acquired to attract or suit specific persons or groups that are not (or hardly) used
	The boys-and-toys effect	Technologies' attractiveness to professionals and patients ("the cool gadget effect")

13.7   Conclusion

In this chapter I have discussed the distinction between utility and futility of technology as well as the question of when to start and when to stop treatment. As emphasized, these issues go to the ethical core of medicine, i.e., to do good and avoid doing harm. Given the vast potential of modern technology, there are ample chances of futile diagnostics and treatment, and modern medicine is extensively charged with doing too much and thereby violating the principles of beneficence, non-maleficence, and justice. The extensive potential of technology also spurs hype, hope, and hubris. To counterbalance such effects and to bar inappropriate technology use in cardiac intensive care units (as in health care in general) we need to identify and address the drivers of excessive technology use. "External" drivers of inappropriate use are related to stakeholders and their roles while "internal" drivers are identified as biases and imperatives in human beings. Both types of drivers can undermine autonomy for patients, professionals, and policy makers deciding on technology in CICU. We need to reflect on and avoid the negative effect of these drivers of medical technology in order to use technology and its great potential to help people in an appropriate way.

References

1. Fisher ES, Welch HG. Avoiding the unintended consequences of growth in medical care: how might more be worse? JAMA. 1999;281:446–53.
2. Curry R. Too much of a good thing: Mae West as cultural icon. Minneapolis: University of Minnesota Press; 1996.
3. Hofmann B. Too much of a good thing is wonderful? A conceptual analysis of excessive examinations and diagnostic futility in diagnostic radiology. Med Health Care Philos. 2010;13:139–48.
4. Luce JM, White DB. A history of ethics and law in the intensive care unit. Crit Care Clin. 2009;25:221–37.
5. Schneiderman LJ, Jecker NS, Jonsen AR. Medical futility: its meaning and ethical implications. Ann Intern Med. 1990;11:949–54.
6. Bernat JL. Medical futility. Neurocrit Care. 2005;2:198–205.
7. Mohindra R. Medical futility: a conceptual model. J Med Ethics. 2007;33:71–5.
8. Moratti S. The development of "medical futility": towards a procedural approach based on the role of the medical profession. J Med Ethics. 2009;35:369–72.
9. Schneiderman LJ. Defining medical futility and improving medical care. J Bioeth Inq. 2011;8:123.
10. Vergano M, Gristina GR. Futility in medicine. Trends Anaesth Crit Care. 2014;4:167–9.
11. Vincent JL. When ICU treatment becomes futile. J Clinic Res Bioeth. 2014;5:1.
12. Aghabarary M, Nayeri ND. Medical futility and its challenges: a review study. J Med Ethics Hist Med. 2016;9:1–13.
13. Šarić L, Prkić I, Jukić M. Futile treatment—a review. J Bioeth Inq. 2017;14:329–37.
14. Morata L. An evolutionary concept analysis of futility in health care. J Adv Nurs. 2018;74:1289–300.
15. Sibbald R, Downar J, Hawryluck L. Perceptions of "futile care" among caregivers in intensive care units. CMAJ. 2007;177:1201–8.
16. Gilligan T, Smith ML, Raffin TA. Ethical issues of care in the cardiac intensive care unit. In: Jeremias A, Brown DL, editors. Cardiac intensive care. 2nd ed. Philadelphia, PA: Sounders Elsevier Inc; 2010. p. 9–24.
17. Wilkinson DJ, Savulescu J. Knowing when to stop: futility in the intensive care unit. Curr Opin Anaesthesiol. 2011;24:160–5.
18. Truog RD, White DB. Futile treatments in intensive care units. JAMA Int Med. 2013;173:1894–5.
19. Huynh TN, Kleerup EC, Raj PP, Wenger NS. The opportunity cost of futile treatment in the intensive care unit. Crit Care Med. 2014;42:1977.
20. Tomlinson T, Brody H. Futility and the ethics of resuscitation. JAMA. 1990;264:1276–80.

21. Kon AA, Shepard EK, Sederstrom NO, Swoboda SM, Marshall MF, Birriel B, et al. Defining futile and potentially inappropriate interventions: a policy statement from the Society of Critical Care Medicine Ethics Committee. Crit Care Med. 2016;44:1769–74.
22. Doty WD, Walker RM. Medical futility. Clin Cardiol. 2000;23(Suppl):6–16.
23. Beauchamp TL, Childress JF. Principles of biomedical ethics. New York: Oxford University Press New York; 2019.
24. Taylor DR, Lightbody CJ. Futility and appropriateness: challenging words, important concepts. Postgrad Med J. 2018;94:238–43.
25. Hofmann B. Overdiagnostic uncertainty. Eur J Epidemiol. 2017;32:533–4.
26. Romanò M. Withholding and withdrawing therapy in cardiac intensive care units: ethical and clinical criteria in end-of-life decisions. G Ital Cardiol. 2011;12:50–7.
27. Romanò M, Gorni G. Implantable cardiac device deactivation at the end of life. G Ital Cardiol. 2020;21:286–95.
28. Romanò M, Piga MA, Bertona R, Negro R, Ruggeri C, Zorzoli F, et al. Implantable cardioverter-defibrillator deactivation at the end of life: Ethical, clinical and communication issues. G Ital Cardiol. 2017;18:139–49.
29. Rothman D. Beginnings count : the technological imperative in American health care. New York: Oxford University Press; 1997.
30. Ursin L. Withholding and withdrawing life-sustaining treatment: ethically equivalent? Amer J Bioeth. 2019;19:10–20.
31. Hofmann B. Categorical mistakes and moral biases in the withholding-versus-withdrawal debate. Amer J Bioeth. 2019;19:29–31.
32. Romanò M. The role of palliative care in the cardiac intensive care unit. Healthcare (Basel). 2019;7:30. https://doi.org/10.3390/healthcare701003033.
33. Romanò M. Facilitating supportive care in cardiac intensive care units. Curr Opin Support Palliat Care. 2020;14:19–24.
34. Richards P. Too much medicine? BMJ. 1999;318:268.
35. Moynihan R, Smith R. Too much medicine? BMJ. 2002;324(7342):859–60.
36. Brownlee S. Overtreated: why too much medicine is making us sicker and poorer. New York: Bloomsbury; 2007.
37. Moynihan R. Too much medicine, not enough mirth. BMJ. 2012;e7116:345.
38. Barraclough K. Too much medicine. Beware the influence of the "SIF" (single issue fanatic) in clinical guidelines. BMJ. 2013;f4719:347.
39. Glasziou P, Moynihan R, Richards T, Godlee F. Too much medicine; too little care. BMJ. 2013;f4247:347.
40. Moynihan R, Glasziou P, Woloshin S, Schwartz L, Santa J, Godlee F. Winding back the harms of too much medicine. BMJ. 2013;f1271:346.
41. Papagiannis A. Too much medicine campaign is long overdue. BMJ. 2013;f1723:346.
42. Welch HG. Less medicine, more health: 7 assumptions that drive too much medical care. Boston, MA: Beacon Press; 2015.
43. Attena F. Too much medicine? Scientific and ethical issues from a comparison between two conflicting paradigms. BMC Public Health. 2019;19:97.
44. Levinson W, Born K, Wolfson D. Choosing wisely campaigns: a work in progress. JAMA. 2018;319:1975–6.
45. Wild C, Mayer J. Overtreatment: Initiatives to identify ineffective and inappropriate medical interventions. Wien Med Wochenschr. 2016;166:149–54.
46. Badgery-Parker T, Pearson S-A, Chalmers K, Brett J, Scott IA, Dunn S, et al. Low-value care in Australian public hospitals: prevalence and trends over time. BMJ Qual Saf. 2019;28:205–14.
47. Colla CH, Morden NE, Sequist TD, Schpero WL, Rosenthal MB. Choosing wisely: prevalence and correlates of low-value health care services in the United States. J Gen Intern Med. 2015;30:221–8.
48. Elshaug AG, Watt AM, Mundy L, Willis CD. Over 150 potentially low-value health care practices: an Australian study. Med J Aust. 2012;197:556–60.
49. McAlister FA, Lin M, Bakal J, Dean S. Frequency of low-value care in Alberta, Canada: a retrospective cohort study. BMJ Qual Saf. 2018;27:340–6.

50. Schwartz AL, Landon BE, Elshaug AG, Chernew ME, McWilliams JM. Measuring low-value care in medicare. JAMA Intern Med. 2014;174:1067–76.
51. Willson A. The problem with eliminating 'low-value care'. BMJ Qual Saf. 2015;24:611–4.
52. Hofmann BM. Too much technology. BMJ. 2015;h705:350.
53. Almeida JPLD, Farias JS, Carvalho HS. Drivers of the technology adoption in healthcare. BBR Braz Bus Rev. 2017;14:336–51.
54. Saini V, Garcia-Armesto S, Klemperer D, Paris V, Elshaug AG, Brownlee S, et al. Drivers of poor medical care. Lancet. 2017;390:178–90.
55. Meskó B. 10 Ways technology is changing healthcare. Future of medicine. The medical futurist; 2020.
56. Hofmann B. Medicalization and overdiagnosis: different but alike. Med Health Care Philos. 2016;19(2):253–64.
57. Hofmann B. Expanding disease and undermining the ethos of medicine. Eur J Epidemiol. 2019;34:613–9.
58. Fryback DG, Thornbury JR. The efficacy of diagnostic imaging. Med Decis Making. 1991;11:88–94.
59. Moynihan R, Heath I, Henry D. Selling sickness: the pharmaceutical industry and disease mongering. BMJ. 2002;324:886–91.
60. Moynihan R, Doran E, Henry D. Disease mongering is now part of the global health debate. PLoS Med. 2008;e106:5.
61. Welch HG, Schwartz L, Woloshin S. Overdiagnosed : making people sick in the pursuit of health. Boston, MA: Beacon Press; 2011. xvii, 228 p.
62. Hermer LD, Brody H. Defensive medicine, cost containment, and reform. J Gen Intern Med. 2010;25:470–3.
63. Berlin L. Medical errors, malpractice, and defensive medicine: an ill-fated triad. Diagnosi. 2017;4:133–9.
64. Kahneman D, Tversky A. Intuitive prediction: biases and corrective procedures. Eugene, Oregon: Decision Research; 1977.
65. Kahneman D, Slovic P, Tversky A. Judgement under uncertainty: heuristics and biases. New York: Cambridge University Press, Cambridge; 1982.
66. Kahneman D, Tversky A. On the reality of cognitive illusions. Psychol Rev. 1996;103:582–91.
67. Hofmann B. Biases distorting priority setting. Health Policy. 2020;124:52–60.
68. Hofmann BM. Categorical mistakes and moral biases in the withholding-versus-withdrawal debate. Am JBioeth. 2019;19(3):29–31.
69. Hofmann BM. Biases and imperatives in handling medical technology. Health Policy Technol. 2019;8:377–85.
70. Hofmann B. Progress bias versus status quo bias in the ethics of emerging science and technology. Bioethics. 2020;34:252–63.
71. Bryan S, Mitton C, Donaldson C. Breaking the addiction to technology adoption. Health Econ. 2014;23:379–83.
72. Niven DJ, Mrklas KJ, Holodinsky JK, Straus SE, Hemmelgarn BR, Jeffs LP. Towards understanding the de-adoption of low-value clinical practices: a scoping review. BMC Med. 2015;13:255.
73. Tymstra T. The imperative character of medical technology and the meaning of "anticipated decision regret". Int J Technol Assess Health Care. 1989;5:207–13.
74. Album D, Johannessen LE, Rasmussen EB. Stability and change in disease prestige: a comparative analysis of three surveys spanning a quarter of a century. Soc Sci Med. 2017;180(1):45–51.
75. Album D, Westin S. Do diseases have a prestige hierarchy? A survey among physicians and medical students. Soc Sci Med. 2008;66(1):182–8.
76. Hofmann B. Biases and imperatives in handling medical technology. Health Policy Technol. 2019: Online Preprint.
77. Mazarr MJ. Rethinking risk in national security: lessons of the financial crisis for risk management. New York: Springer; 2016.
78. Chatterjee K. The Swan-Ganz catheters: past, present, and future. Circulation. 2009;119(1):147–52.

Physician Education and Training in Palliative Care: A New Challenge in Modern Cardiac Intensive Care

Elizabeth Sonntag, Emily Rivet, Jason Katz, Danielle Noreika, and Evgenia Granina

14.1 Introduction: The Modern Cardiac Intensive Care Unit

After its introduction into the framework for medical care in the 1960s, the coronary care unit (CCU) spread rapidly throughout the country and became established within contemporary healthcare systems as a validated means for improving outcomes for patients with acute myocardial infarction (MI) [1]. Today's CCU, however, looks very different from these pioneer units, and instead is home to an increasingly diverse population of patients with advanced critical illness, complicating a multitude of cardiovascular conditions. To reflect the fact that these units are

E. Sonntag (✉)
Department of Internal Medicine, Division of Pulmonary and Critical Care Medicine,
Virginia Commonwealth University, Richmond, VA, USA
e-mail: Elizabeth.Sonntag@vcuhealth.org

E. Rivet
Department of Surgery, Division of Colon and Rectal Surgery, Virginia Commonwealth
University, Richmond, VA, USA
e-mail: Emily.Rivet@vcuhealth.org

J. Katz
Department of Internal Medicine, Division of Cardiology, Duke University,
Durham, NC, USA
e-mail: jason.katz@duke.edu

D. Noreika
Department of Internal Medicine, Division of Hematology, Oncology & Palliative Care,
Virginia Commonwealth University, Richmond, VA, USA
e-mail: danielle.noreika@vcuhealth.org

E. Granina
Hospice and Palliative Care Fellowship, Virginia Commonwealth University,
Richmond, VA, USA
e-mail: Evgenia.Granina@vcuhealth.org

M. Romanò (ed.), *Palliative Care in Cardiac Intensive Care Units*,
https://doi.org/10.1007/978-3-030-80112-0_14

"

truly home to complex critically ill patients, many have adopted a new moniker for these care environments: the cardiac intensive care unit (CICU). Patients that occupy the modern CICU have more comorbidities and greater illness severity and leverage more critical care resources than ever before. Those with acute MI are now often the minority, replaced instead by patients with all forms of shock, multisystem organ failure, electrical storm, valvular emergencies, end-stage heart failure, and other unstable clinical conditions. An increasing population of CICU patients require life-support modalities typically only available in an intensive care setting, including vasopressors, inotropic agents, invasive mechanical ventilation, and continuous renal replacement therapies. Additionally, the use of mechanical circulatory support (MCS) technologies—including intra-aortic balloon pumps, temporary axial and centrifugal flow pumps, surgically implanted left ventricular assist devices (LVADs), and extracorporeal membrane oxygenation (ECMO)—has become commonplace [2]. A growing body of evidence has now substantiated the notion that patients within the modern CICU are sicker and at greater risk for mortality than ever before [3]. The epidemiology and patterns of care in the modern CICUs are discussed in detail in Chap. 1.

The majority of high-volume CICUs can be found within academic or university-based hospitals, and therefore are teaching environments for learners at multiple levels of training including medical students, residents, and fellows. Though walking a patient and family through difficult prognosis, adjustment to new therapies, symptom management, and end-of-life care is the commonplace for CICU providers, there is currently no formal curriculum for palliative care in internal medicine or cardiology training. Rather than relying on palliative care consultation services at the end of life, primary palliative care should be considered for all patients managed in a CICU and/or receiving life-prolonging therapy. However, the question remains as to what to teach and how to best teach it. This chapter discusses the challenge of cardiac intensive care physician education and training in palliative care. Though more research is needed in order to figure out how best to implement primary palliative care education for providers in the CICU, this chapter identifies major tenants of primary palliative care, learning objectives for practicing primary palliative care, and teaching modalities which will best serve these learning objectives.

14.2 Palliative Care in the CICU

Palliative care is a specialty that focuses on the quality of life, relief of suffering, psychosocial and spiritual needs, and alignment of treatments with care goals for patients with serious illness [4]. As the patient population in the CICU has evolved, palliative care has become increasingly relevant due to the severity and complexity of conditions managed in these units. Of note, patients with cardiovascular disease represent the largest disease group in need of palliative care at the end of life [5]. Given the high mortality of heart failure patients (40% die within 1 year of their first hospitalization) and the recommendation of several societies, including the American College of Cardiology, the American Heart Association, the International

Society for Heart and Lung Transplantation, and the Heart Failure Society of America, many programs have integrated palliative care into their management of advanced heart failure patients, and particularly those supported by LVADs [6]. Furthermore, the Centers for Medicare and Medicaid Services and the Joint Commission require that a palliative care specialist be a part of the core multidisciplinary MCS team [7]. Several organizations such as the Heart Failure Working Group of the Danish Society of Cardiology and the Heart Failure Association of the European Society of Cardiology have published position statements on palliative care in the heart failure patient population that include advocacy for early intervention, clarification of the role of palliative care, and guidelines for conversations about device deactivation [8]. The American Heart Association and the American Stroke Association put forth a joint statement in 2016 that describes the benefits of palliative care and emphasizes the importance of both primary palliative care performed by the cardiac interdisciplinary team and access to specialty palliative care [9]. One systematic review and meta-analysis suggested that palliative care is associated with improved quality of life and reduced symptom burden [10]. In the Palliative Care in Heart Failure trial (2017) the palliative care intervention arm (usual care plus a 6-month interdisciplinary palliative care intervention) was associated with clinically significant improvements in quality of life as well as improvements in mood (anxiety and depression) and spiritual well-being, compared to usual care alone [11]. Palliative care has also been shown to be beneficial in intensive care settings. For example, early involvement of palliative care leads to earlier family meetings and decreased hospital length of stay [12]. Involvement of palliative care also improves alignment of treatment decisions with patient's values and preferences [13]. Combining this evidence supports that the tenants of palliative care should be familiar to the physicians offering and managing advanced cardiac care.

14.3   Primary and Specialty Palliative Care in the CICU

Palliative care can be provided through several paradigms. The first, often termed "primary palliative care," refers to the delivery of palliative care by the treating team caring for the patient [14]. In the CICU environment, this would generally be the CICU intensivists. Primary palliative care is defined as the provision of basic palliative care components by clinicians who are not formally trained in specialty palliative care (of note, this can include physicians, advanced practice providers, nurses, social workers, and other interdisciplinary team members). There is no research to guide the optimal approach to integrating primary palliative care in subspecialty practices, so there remains individual variability in incorporation [15]. There are a number of skills that could be included in training clinicians in primary palliative care. In a recent publication by an embedded palliative care service in a tertiary care heart failure center, symptom management and care planning were the two most common reasons for referral. The most common symptoms managed were pain, anorexia, insomnia, depression, and anxiety, and opioids were the most commonly prescribed medication. Shared care planning, code status, and hospice were the most commonly discussed care planning topics [16]. Other topics that may be relevant to primary palliative skills within cardiology include discussions regarding the use of advanced cardiac therapies such as chronic inotropes, mechanical ventilation, implantable cardioverter-defibrillators (ICDs), pacemakers, MCS, therapeutic hypothermia, and cardiac transplantation. Although recognized as important to their patient population, only 10% of cardiologists in one survey reported formal education in palliative care during their cardiovascular training [17].

Alternatively, "specialty" palliative care can be performed by a separate multidisciplinary team which generally includes a provider with advanced training and certification in Hospice and Palliative Medicine as well as experts in fields such as social work and chaplaincy. Because the availability of formally trained palliative care providers is limited, the introduction of palliative care concepts and the promotion of primary palliative care skill sets for CICU team members are vital. As the majority of high-volume CICUs are located within academic or university-based hospital systems, access to specialty palliative care is often available although it cannot be assumed. However, the ability of CICU intensivists to provide primary palliative care as exemplified by familiarity with the basic principles of palliative care is important for several reasons. Specialty palliative care is a limited resource and may be challenging to access acutely. Furthermore, palliative care is relevant to so many aspects of patient care in the CICU, as the life-sustaining technologies employed in the CICU often have significant implications for quality of life, healthcare decision-making, and end-of-life care. Therefore, it is ideal to integrate these skills into basic practice. As such, there is an opportunity to enhance knowledge and skills in experienced CICU clinicians by considering their work through the lens of palliative care.

14.4 Physician Education and Training

Primary palliative care education is not yet compulsory in undergraduate medical education or graduate medical education and therefore varies widely across institutions. In a review of the scope of training in medical residencies and fellowships, primary palliative care teaching emphasized communication and symptom management topics with instruction via didactics. Most of the time, the assessed outcome was attitude. Internal medicine was among one of the residencies most represented, but cardiology fellowship or heart failure fellowship programs were not. In a review of internal medicine residency programs, the most common domains studied included communication, symptom management, end of life, psychological support, transition of care or resources, ethics, and bereavement. The most common methods of teaching included didactics or lectures, discussion, rotations, workshops or retreats, simulation/role play, standardized patients, independent learning, and Web-based learning. Residents were measured on outcomes such as subjective knowledge, objective knowledge, attitudes, and observation of skills. Most residency and fellowship programs that were included in a recent survey reported little to no directed palliative care didactics and training. For example, cardiology fellowship had none [18]. Objectives of physician education and training in palliative care include provider understanding the clinical indications of therapies unique to the CICU, followed by mastering primary palliative care skills such as communication, decision-making, and symptom management. Teaching modalities that best serve this mission include bedside teaching, case-based teaching, and didactics.

14.5 Primary Palliative Care Learning Objectives

The Accreditation Counsel for Graduate Medical Education (ACGME) and the American College of Cardiology (ACC) have set forth training requirements which include palliative care for those pursuing fellowships in cardiology and advanced heart failure. Despite these recommendations one group of researchers surveyed cardiology fellows and found that although 71% reported clinical collaboration with palliative care specialists during training, less than 10% had received formal education in palliative care topics [19]. Therefore, physicians who practice in the CICU setting are often not expert in providing palliative care [20]. On the contrary, fellowships in palliative care medicine provide extensive training over the course of 1 year, with a focus on skills for enhancing patient quality of life, reducing symptom burden related to severe illness, and supporting patients and their loved ones through the dying process [21]. Many areas of palliative care training are applicable to the care of patients in the CICU and can guide the objectives for learning primary palliative care in the CICU (Table 14.1). This section has broken down primary palliative care learning objectives into three main categories: communication, decision-making, and symptom management.

14.6 Communication

Patients in the CICU are critically ill, medically complex, and often near the end of their life. Therefore, clear and empathetic communication is vital, and effective communication should be taught to all providers caring for patients in the CICU.

Communication skills important early on in a patient encounter include displaying empathy, building relationships and trust with a patient and/or their proxies, and setting expectations. It is important for a provider to develop a relationship with a patient/family at the beginning of the CICU admission, rather than waiting for the goals of care discussion at a time of patient decompensation or high stress. As a patient progresses and prognosis becomes more clear, CICU providers must have skills to translate complicated diagnoses, treatment plans, and prognoses to patients and proxies in an individualized way such that it is understandable to the recipient. As a patient's primary provider, they must also be able to organize and summarize recommendations made by consultants and other members of the multidisciplinary CICU team. Practicing of specific skills, such as "breaking bad news" and "leading goals of care discussions," will be vital in a provider's comfort and proficiency in CICU communication. When discussing goals of care, it is imperative that the

Table 14.1 Primary palliative care learning objectives for cardiac intensive care unit providers

Communication Provider must be proficient in effective communication	Decision-making Provider must be skilled in decision-making		Symptom management Provider must be able to relieve suffering, both physical and emotional
Displaying empathy	**Prognostication** Clinical judgement	**Shared decision-making** Patient and family-centered decision-making	Pain assessment and management
Relationship and trust building	Effective application of life-sustaining therapy	Taking part in active shared decision-making	Dyspnea assessment and management
Expectation setting	Making recommendations in the face of uncertainty	Eliciting patient values and preferences	Delirium assessment and management
Translation of complex medical diagnosis, treatment plan, and prognosis	Understanding limitations of life-sustaining therapy	Balancing benefit and burden of treatment options	Sleep disturbance assessment and management
Summarize recommendations of consultants	Withholding potentially inappropriate therapy	Respect diversity in attitude, religion, and culture	Anxiety and depression assessment and management
Breaking bad news	Transitioning goals of care	Capacity assessment	Comfort in transitioning from full support to comfort care, including withdrawal of life-sustaining therapy
Leading goals-of-care discussions	Recognizing patients who may benefit from hospice referral	Advance care planning	Ability to emotionally and practically support family or other caregivers through bereavement
Eliciting patient values and preferences		Guiding surrogate through decision-making using substituted judgment	Understanding when to refer to specialty palliative care
Managing requests for potentially inappropriate therapy			
Comforting the bereaved			

[20, 32, 33, 6, 34]

provider is comfortable eliciting the values and preferences of the patient; engaging in discussions regarding spirituality, religion, and cultural expectations; and managing requests for potentially inappropriate therapy. Finally, communication around death and dying, including comforting for the bereaved, is an important skill. These communication skills are crucial for guiding patients and/or their proxies through the decision-making process.

14.7 Decision-Making

Complex decisions must be made in the CICU setting, often in the face of uncertainty, which first requires the beneficent provider to have expert clinical and prognostic judgment. Then, in order to best uphold a patient's autonomy, providers must be prepared to practice shared decision-making.

Critical care practice requires the ability to deftly navigate between highly specialized recovery-directed care and recognition of the limits of this care, to then empathetically facilitate a transition to care focused on comfort. Vital to this is gaining skills in prognostication. Accurate prognostication allows for effective application of life-sustaining therapies such as MCS, vasopressors, inotropes, ventilator, and continuous veno-venous hemodialysis, so that it is in-line with goals of care and will serve the expected outcome. When this is not possible, the provider should be prepared to make recommendations in the face of uncertainty. Though recovery is a primary goal, understanding the limitations of life-sustaining therapy is of the utmost importance. CICU providers must understand not only clinical indications, but also the limitations of intensive therapies, and when to withhold potentially inappropriate and/or life-sustaining therapies while instead guiding families through the dying process. It is important for CICU providers to identify patients who may qualify for and benefit from hospice.

14.8 Therapies and Interventions Unique to CICU

First, it will be important for trainees to understand clinical indications related to life-sustaining therapies and CICU care such as MCS, vasopressors, inotropes, ventilator, and dialysis. They will need to be expert in prognostication. Thoroughly grasping the clinical indications for particular treatments is the first step in being able to counsel patients/proxies as to whether the therapy will serve the goals of care. Understanding the limitations of these therapies will aid in avoiding potentially inappropriate interventions. Advanced therapies used in the CICU are discussed in detail in Chap. 2. Furthermore limitations to advanced therapies, including deactivation of implanted cardiac devices, and withholding and withdrawal of life-sustaining therapy, are discussed in Chaps. 6, 7, 8, and 10.

14.9 Shared Decision-Making

Shared decision-making is imperative in applying the above therapies to care in the CICU. Shared decision-making is the way by which providers and patients make healthcare decisions that best align with the patient's wishes and respect their autonomy. In this construct the provider must first elicit the patient's values and preferences, and then use their medical judgement to balance benefits and burdens of a particular plan of care and advise which treatment plan is most likely to achieve the patient's desired goals. Shared decision-making and advanced directives are discussed in detail in Chap. 5.

14.10 Symptom Management

Evaluating and managing symptoms are core aspects of both primary and specialty palliative care. Patients with inadequately managed symptoms (including pain or dyspnea) cannot be expected to benefit from other elements of palliative care such as participation in conversations directed at healthcare decision-making. As such, an important step in providing palliative care is to assess for symptoms. As previously mentioned, acute or decompensated heart failure is a common reason for admission to the CICU. Similar to other advanced disease states and the failure of other organs, patients with heart failure may experience a range of symptoms including dyspnea, fatigue, pain, loss of appetite, insomnia, and cough [22]. Psychiatric and cognitive dysfunction including delirium is also common [23]. The trajectory of decline in cardiac failure is notable for its lack of predictability and is characterized by sudden decompensations followed by periods of remission [24]. During these decompensations, providers practicing in the CICU should be prepared to address symptoms such as pain, dyspnea, fatigue, and delirium. A detailed review related to evaluation and management of symptoms is provided in Chap. 3 of this text, and should be used as a resource for education.

14.11 Teaching Modalities

Common clinical teaching methods are listed in Table 14.2 and include bedside teaching, didactics, and case-based teaching. Whenever possible, the teaching of primary palliative care in the CICU should be taught by a palliative care physician or a critical care physician comfortable with palliative care and CICU care.

14.12 Bedside Teaching

Bedside teaching is a core tenant of medical education. It can be an effective mode of teaching communication through role-modeling, decision-making through mentorship, and symptom management via experience with bedside cases.

Table 14.2 Methods of teaching

Bedside		Didactics		Case based	
Teaching method	Goals	Teaching method	Goals	Teaching method	Goals
Role-modeling	Learner participates in goals-of-care discussions, family meetings, and sessions in which shared decision-making will occur, and learns communication skills via observation of expert	Lecture	Learner is introduced to topics that will be encountered during bedside management of patients and has the opportunity to ask questions and seek clarification in order to grow their fund of knowledge	Case review	Learner reviews a case allowing time for discussion of and reasoning through plan of care and communication strategies
Mentorship	Learner leads goals-of-care discussions, family meetings, and sessions in which shared decision-making will occur, and gets feedback on communication skills Learner receives feedback on plan of care and symptom management strategies	Targeted reading/ journal club	Learner reviews literature that will guide evidence-based practice and grow their fund of knowledge	Simulation	Learner is able to practice communication skills
Palliative care rotation	Learner gains experience in primary palliative care via exposure to a larger number of patients with end-of-life and/or symptom management needs				

[29, 31]

Role-modeling and mentorship are important factors, especially for resident and fellow learning. Most CICU physicians will not go on to receive specialized training in hospice and palliative medicine; therefore, improvement of primary palliative care skills often depends on the accumulation of personal experience and observation of successful strategies demonstrated by other providers. Attending physicians should role model communication by allowing learners to take part in goals of care discussions, breaking bad news, and shared decision-making, and then be prepared to mentor learners via giving guidance, support, and feedback. For example, following the timeless "see one, do one, teach one" model of medicine, learners should have opportunities to witness well-executed primary palliative care by an experienced provider. They should then practice leading the delivery of that care, and/or goals of care discussions with opportunities for feedback. Finally, when proficient in skill and comfort, learners should teach primary palliative care to others. Learners will also benefit via firsthand experience in caring for patients who require primary palliative care—this can be undertaken on a palliative care rotation where they can be mentored by palliative care experts, or through co-managing patient care in the CICU. Learners benefit when expert CICU clinicians role-model communcation and palliaitve care skills; however, expertise may vary from provider to provider. Therefore, training should ensure that there are didactic and case-based educational opportunities to supplement bedside teaching.

14.13 Didactics

Didactic education is aimed at improving the learner's fund of knowledge and typically consists of lectures and target reading. When surveyed, non-palliative care providers who were asked about primary palliative care education mostly preferred didactic lectures for education when offered options that also included online curriculum, retreats, "coaching" during patient care, standardized patient encounters, and audio review of patient encounters [25]. Didactic teaching lends itself well to the teaching of symptom management. Although symptom management in palliative care is often most commonly ascribed to cancer patients, it has been shown that symptoms are common in a number of other life-limiting illnesses including cardiac diseases such as heart failure [26]. There are a number of symptoms that palliative patients with underlying life-limiting illnesses can experience that may need to be evaluated and managed including but not limited to pain, dyspnea, nausea, anxiety, depression, anorexia, insomnia, constipation/diarrhea, and fatigue. Effective symptom management starts with assessment which can be introduced in a didactic setting prior to modeling in actual patient encounters. In addition to serving as a mechanism for providing education to teams caring for patients with advanced cardiac illnesses, didactic lectures can create a forum to encourage awareness of system resources for assistance in symptom management or advance care planning in these patients. Despite the importance of didactics, a survey from 2020 on residency and fellowship programs found varied uptake on palliative didactic topics including multiple training programs that had none at all [18]. Therefore, the implementation of primary palliative care didactics into the teaching of primary palliative care in the CICU is an important target.

14.14 Case Based

The American Heart Association and the American College of Cardiology, Core Cardiology Training Symposium (ACC COCATS) make recommendations for competencies cardiologists should achieve during training. For example, the cardiology trainee must master communication and exhibit empathy and compassion while becoming comfortable with leading family meetings, including those that discuss goals of care and end-of-life issues. Despite these recommendations most trainees do not undergo any formal training. Case-based learning often works to reinforce didactic teaching. In contrast to traditional lecture-based teaching (which is passive) new methods of teaching that are learner centered and promote active learning have been beneficial to medical education. Using active learning for the development of communication skills is particularly beneficial for teaching primary palliative care [27]. There are also opportunities to incorporate role-playing, videos of best practice, and simulation into educational programs. Case-based teaching lends itself well to teaching palliative care, as it is learner centered, and allows more time to be spent on working through problems and discussing viewpoints. In addition simulation of cases (for example goals-of-care discussions or breaking bad news) may help a learner practice valuable communication skills in a safe environment, before interacting with a patient, and has been shown to help learners retain skills and knowledge [28]. Learners may even benefit from attending an outside workshop or retreat. VitalTalk [29] offers evidence-based curriculum to improve communication skills surrounding serious illness. It has been shown to improve skills in specialties such as oncology, nephrology, and geriatrics. A group out of the University of Pittsburgh Medical Center health system designed a workshop called CardioTalk (molded after VitalTalk) which was aimed at imparting valuable communication skills specifically around challenging conversations for providers who practice in the cardiac intensive care unit [30]. First-year cardiology fellows and cardiology attendings participated in a 2+ days' workshop which included didactics and simulated patient encounters, followed by some small group conversations around observations and feedback. This training was well received by both the fellows and the attendings who took the course. All of the learners had a statistically significant increase in perceived preparedness for the following skills: giving bad news, running a family meeting, expressing empathy, discussing treatment options, negotiating denial, discussing withdrawal of treatment, request for futile treatment, discussion of code status, discussion of spiritual concerns, and family end-of-life concerns [31].

14.15 Conclusion

Primary palliative care should be taught to all providers in the CICU. A combination of teaching modalities, including bedside teaching, didactics, and case-based teaching, should be deployed to ensure that learners understand the clinical indications of therapies and interventions unique to the CICU, obtain key communication skills, can navigate complex decision-making, and are proficient in symptom management.

References

1. Loughran J, Puthawala T, Sutton BS, Brown LE, Pronovost PJ, DeFilippis AP. The cardiovascular intensive care unit—an evolving model for health care delivery. J Intensive Care Med. 2017;32(2):116–23.
2. Katz JN, Minder M, Olenchock B, Price S, Goldfarb M, Washam JB, et al. The genesis, maturation, and future of critical care cardiology. J Am Coll Cardiol. 2016;68(1):67–79.
3. Kasaoka S. Evolved role of the cardiovascular intensive care unit (CICU). J Intensive Care [Internet]. 2017 Dec 22 [cited 2021 Jan 11];5. Available from: https://www.ncbi.nlm.nih.gov/pmc/articles/PMC5741934/
4. Palliative Care [Internet]. [cited 2021 Jan 11]. Available from: https://www.who.int/news-room/fact-sheets/detail/palliative-care
5. Sullivan AM, Lakoma MD, Billings JA, Peters AS, Block SD. PCEP Core Faculty. Teaching and learning end-of-life care: evaluation of a faculty development program in palliative care. Acad Med. 2005;80(7):657–68.
6. Kavalieratos D, Gelfman LP, Tycon LE, Riegel B, Bekelman DB, Ikejiani D, et al. Integration of palliative care in heart failure: rationale, evidence, and future priorities. J Am Coll Cardiol. 2017;70(15):1919–30.
7. Wordingham SE, McIlvennan CK. Palliative care for patients on mechanical circulatory support. AMA J Ethics. 2019;21(5):435–42.
8. Jaarsma T, Beattie JM, Ryder M, Rutten FH, McDonagh T, Mohacsi P, et al. Palliative care in heart failure: a position statement from the palliative care workshop of the Heart Failure Association of the European Society of Cardiology. Eur J Heart Fail. 2009; 11(5):433–43.
9. Braun LT, Grady KL, Kutner JS, Adler E, Berlinger N, Boss R, et al. Palliative care and cardiovascular disease and stroke: a policy statement from the American Heart Association/American Stroke Association. Circulation. 2016;134(11):e198–225.
10. Xie K, Gelfman L, Horton JR, Goldstein NE. State of research on palliative care in heart failure as evidenced by published literature, conference proceedings, and NIH Funding. J Card Fail. 2017;23(2):197–200.
11. Rogers JG, Patel CB, Mentz RJ, Granger BB, Steinhauser KE, Fiuzat M, et al. Palliative care in heart failure: the PAL-HF randomized, Controlled Clinical Trial. J Am Coll Cardiol. 2017;70(3):331–41.
12. Mercadante S, Gregoretti C, Cortegiani A. Palliative care in intensive care units: why, where, what, who, when, how. BMC Anesthesiol. 2018;18(1):106.
13. Wordingham SE, McIlvennan CK, Fendler TJ, Behnken AL, Dunlay SM, Kirkpatrick JN, et al. Palliative care clinicians caring for patients before and after continuous flow-left ventricular assist device. J Pain Symptom Manage. 2017;54(4):601–8.
14. Ernecoff NC, Check D, Bannon M, Hanson LC, Dionne-Odom JN, Corbelli J, et al. Comparing specialty and primary palliative care interventions: analysis of a systematic review. J Palliat Med. 2019;23(3):389–96.

15. Quill TE, Abernethy AP. Generalist plus specialist palliative care—creating a more sustainable model. N Engl J Med. 2013;368(13):1173–5.
16. Gandesbery B, Dobbie K, Gorodeski EZ. Outpatient palliative cardiology service embedded within a heart failure clinic: experiences with an emerging model of care. Am J Hosp Palliat Care. 2018;35(4):635–9.
17. Kirkpatrick JN, Hauptman PJ, Swetz KM, Blume ED, Gauvreau K, Maurer M, et al. Palliative care for patients with end-stage cardiovascular disease and devices: a report from the palliative care working group of the geriatrics section of the American College of Cardiology. JAMA Intern Med. 2016;176(7):1017–9.
18. Spiker M, Paulsen K, Mehta AK. Primary palliative care education in U.S. residencies and fellowships: a systematic review of program leadership perspectives. J Palliat Med. 2020;23(10):1392–9.
19. Crousillat Daniela R, Keeley Brieze R, Zheng Hui R, Polk Donna M, Buss Mary K, Schaefer Kristen G. Abstract 18451: palliative care education in cardiology: a national survey of fellows and faculty. Circulation. 2017;136(suppl_1):A18451.
20. DeVita MA, Arnold RM, Barnard D. Teaching palliative care to critical care medicine trainees. Crit Care Med. 2003;31(4):1257–62.
21. 2020 Accreditation Council for Graduate Medical Education (ACGME). ACGME program requirements for graduate medical education in hospice and palliative medicine [Internet]. 2020. Available from: https://www.acgme.org/Portals/0/PFAssets/ProgramRequirements/540_HospicePalliativeMedicine_2020.pdf?ver=2020-06-29-164052-453
22. Lowey SE. Palliative care in the management of patients with advanced heart failure. Adv Exp Med Biol. 2018;1067:295–311.
23. Kida K, Doi S, Suzuki N. Palliative care in patients with advanced heart failure. Heart Fail Clin. 2020;16(2):243–54.
24. Goldstein NE, Lynn J. Trajectory of end-stage heart failure: the influence of technology and implications for policy change. Perspect Biol Med. 2006;49(1):10–8.
25. Carroll T, Weisbrod N, O'Connor A, Quill T. Primary palliative care education: a pilot survey. Am J Hosp Palliat Care. 2018;35(4):565–9.
26. Kelley AS, Morrison RS. Palliative care for the seriously ill. N Engl J Med. 2015;373(8):747–55. Campion EW, editor.
27. Mourad A, Jurjus A, Hajj Hussein I. The what or the how: a review of teaching tools and methods in medical education. MedSciEduc. 2016;26(4):723–8.
28. Boland JW, Barclay S, Gibbins J. Twelve tips for developing palliative care teaching in an undergraduate curriculum for medical students. Med Teach. 2019;41(12):1359–65.
29. Home [Internet]. VitalTalk. [cited 2021 Feb 11]. Available from: https://www.vitaltalk.org/
30. ESC Cardio Talk—The ESC Podcast [Internet]. [cited 2021 Feb 11]. Available from: https://www.escardio.org/The-ESC/What-we-do/news/ESC-Cardio-Talk
31. Berlacher K, Arnold RM, Reitschuler-Cross E, Teuteberg J, Teuteberg W. The impact of communication skills training on cardiology fellows' and attending physicians' perceived comfort with difficult conversations. J Palliat Med. 2017;20(7):767–9.
32. Mularski RA, Curtis JR, Billings JA, Burt R, Byock I, Fuhrman C, et al. Proposed quality measures for palliative care in the critically ill: a consensus from the Robert Wood Johnson Foundation Critical Care Workgroup. Crit Care Med. 2006;34(11 Suppl):S404–11.
33. Danis M, Federman D, Fins JJ, Fox E, Kastenbaum B, Lanken PN, et al. Incorporating palliative care into critical care education: principles, challenges, and opportunities. Crit Care Med. 1999;27(9):2005–13.
34. Crousillat DR, Keeley BR, Buss MK, Zheng H, Polk DM, Schaefer KG. Palliative care education in cardiology. J Am Coll Cardiol. 2018;71(12):1391–4.

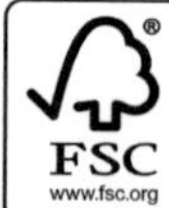

If you have any concerns about our products,
you can contact us on
ProductSafety@springernature.com

In case Publisher is established outside the EU,
the EU authorized representative is:
**Springer Nature Customer Service Center GmbH
Europaplatz 3, 69115 Heidelberg, Germany**

Printed by Libri Plureos GmbH
in Hamburg, Germany